Baby at the Table

A 3-step guide to weaning the Italian way

Michela *and* Emanuela Chiappa

MICHAEL JOSEPH
an imprint of
Penguin Books

MICHAEL JOSEPH

UK | USA | Canada | Ireland | Australia

India | New Zealand | South Africa

Michael Joseph is part of the Penguin Random House group of companies

whose addresses can be found at global.penguinrandomhouse.com.

 Penguin
Random House
UK

Set in Amasis MT Pro, Avenir and Yard Sale

Colour reproduction by Born Group

Printed in Italy by Printer Trento

A CIP catalogue record for this book is available from the British Library

ISBN: 978-0-718-18294-6

www.greenpenguin.co.uk

Penguin Random House is committed to a
sustainable future for our business, our readers
and our planet. This book is made from Forest
Stewardship Council® certified paper.

CONTENTS

OUR PHILOSOPHY

To an Italian, food is a way of life, not just a necessity. The kitchen table should be a place where a family cooks, eats and interacts as one unit... and the heartbeat of every child's upbringing.

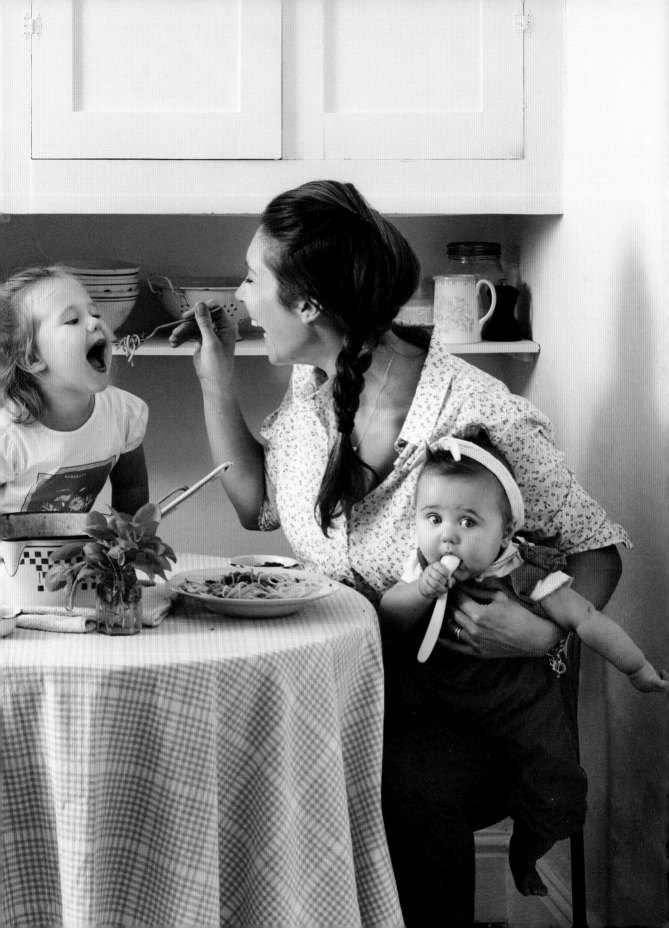

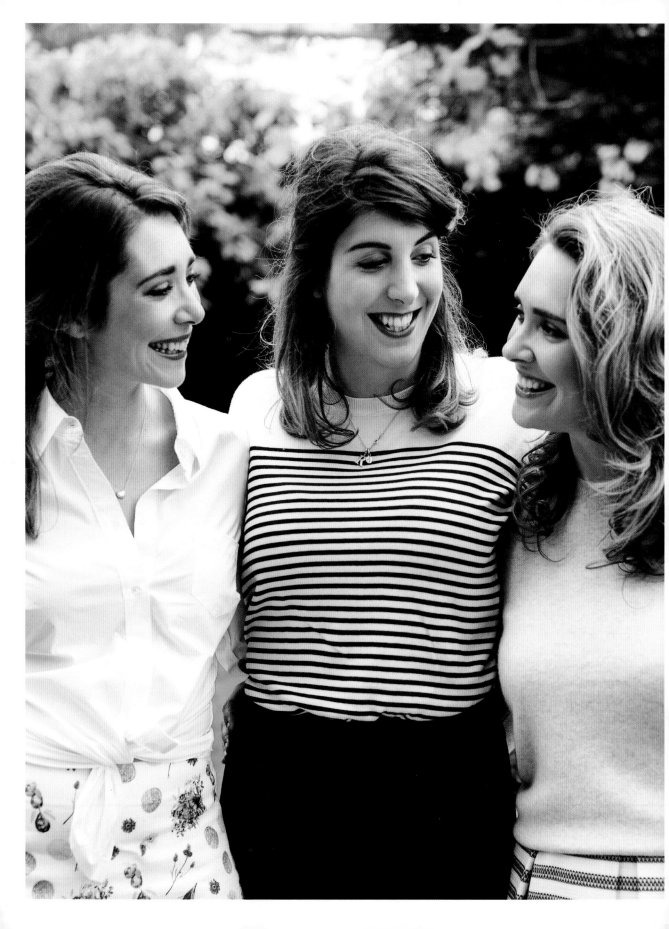

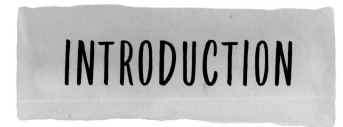

INTRODUCTION

Italians live to eat, and this is certainly how we've been raised. We were in the kitchen from birth, eating and tasting everything. We were always involved in some way, whether it was simply interacting socially while our mum cooked, making lots of mess with flour and eggs, or helping out with the meals when we were a bit older.

Those of you who know me and my sisters, Emi and Romina, will be aware that we have been raised in a large Italian community in South Wales. Brought up in an Italian brood, we lived next door to our uncle, aunt, cousins and grandparents, so our lives have been hugely influenced by both the Italian and the British ways of living, and our upbringing has been focused on family and food.

Emi and I have recently become first-time mums. Fiamma was two years old when I gave birth to Serafina, and Emi added another girl to the clan when she had Fiorenza.

It has been our mission to retain as many Italian values and traditions as possible and to encourage our children to become interested in food from the start. We cherish any recipes and tips our mum raised us on and want to pass them on to you to make weaning your baby and cooking for the family simple and practical.

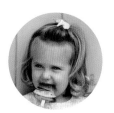

Fiamma: *2 years old. Loves fresh ravioli in brodo, kiwi (with the skin on), watermelon, salmon and nuts. Does not like cherry tomatoes, but will devour raspberries at lightning speed.*

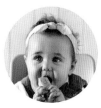

Serafina: *7 months. Mad about beetroot and anything she can get her teeth into (a dried apricot or pineapple core will keep her entertained for at least 20 minutes!).*

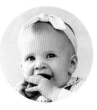

Fiorenza: *10 months. A true carnivore – add any meat to a purée and she will devour it in seconds. Loves blueberries and sweetcorn, but refuses to eat beetroot [no matter how disguised it is in food].*

Every parent will be able to live by this philosophy, no matter how little time they have. However, we know it's easy to make excuses. Maybe you find yourself saying:

'I just don't have the time to cook fresh food every day.'

'My kids are picky and I can't get them to eat the same meals as us.'

'I'm too tired to cook. I forgot to make it to the shops, so the kids will have to make do.'

If so, this book is for you!

Yes, our lives today are busier. We are a society of mega multi-taskers and we all strive to be high fliers in every aspect of life; we want the successful career alongside the dream partner and a great social life, while juggling a family and being a textbook parent. But the reality is often different, and this means that cooking can be side-tracked in favour of supermarket sweeps and a quick-fix microwave meal or 'healthy' and expensive organic meal deals.

I've spoken to mums who tell me that they were obsessed with cooking fresh and delicious meals for their firstborn, but now that they have more kids they 'make do', or cook the same things over and over again, as they can't handle tantrums or picky eaters.

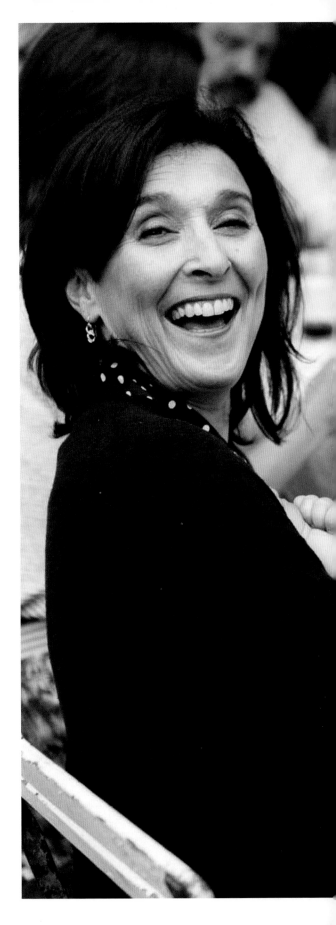

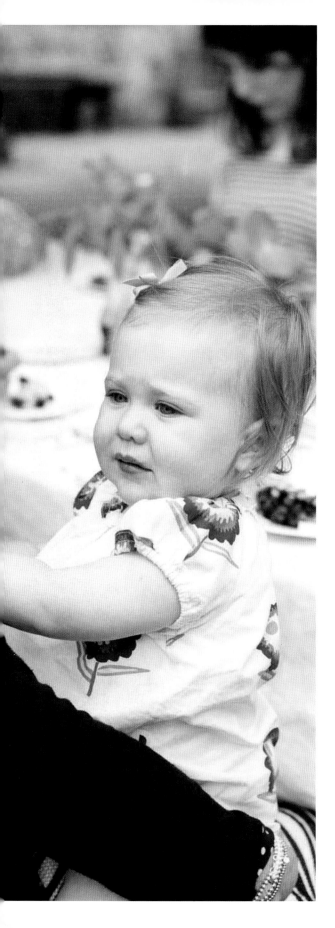

Time for change...

Food and family should be at the heart of what we do. Eating well is not just important for our health, it's what makes the world go round. In our opinion, this food education should start from birth.

We should stop treating kids differently.

Why can't a six-year-old enjoy scallops or fresh porcini with garlic?

Why should they be given a kids' meal?

As for cooking three different meals at three different times for babies, kids and adults – stop right there! Yes, there could be reasons why families think that's easier to manage, but the knock-on effect of this will be felt later in life.

So what to do? How can we get baby weaned and eating fresh meals from scratch, while sitting at the table with the rest of the family, in as little time as possible?

That's where *Baby at the Table* comes in. Emi and I have put all our experiences and recipes into this book, in order to help any parent who wants to try to cook fresh family meals every day while juggling all those other balls that get thrown at them.

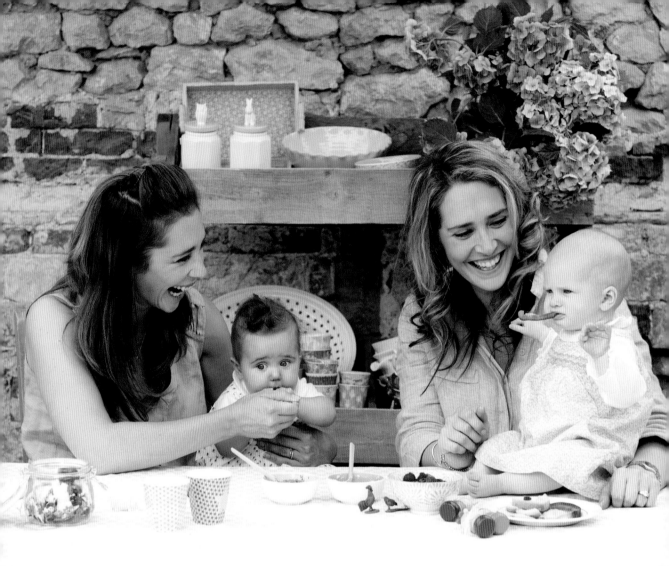

WHY WE'VE WRITTEN THIS BOOK

My sisters and I were brought up in the Welsh valleys, in an
Italian household in which our mum and grandmother were
housewives. The focus was providing food for the family, and
it centred around the philosophy of 'one family, one meal'.

We, on the other hand, are not housewives and have busy lives centred around our careers. However, having had such strong values instilled in us, we have been determined to continue this way of life alongside our careers. So we started adapting traditional recipes and methods in order that we can still cook and eat like Italians, while juggling the other roles we have taken on.

Practical, quick, nutritious solutions for busy parents

Our aim is to share our experiences, tips and recipes in order to help any busy parent cook delicious meals for the whole family. I believe that if you start when your children are young (as early as the weaning stage), you can prevent them turning into picky eaters down the line and raise them to appreciate and value good food.

The following pages contain some of the ideas that have worked for Emi and me, giving you a simple but practical guide to weaning. Using the ABC Weaning Steps (see page 54), by the age of 1 your baby should be eating a version of the same meal you create for your family.

The majority of the recipes have a preparation time of less than 15 minutes – do-able for even the time-poor parent.

Possible? Absolutely!

We have included all our favourite family recipes and tweaked them so most of them have a preparation time of less than 15 minutes. We've also included some clever tips and tricks to help you out along the way.

We want to help busy parents produce simple, nutritious meals around a busy schedule and encourage their babies to eat healthy, home-cooked food.

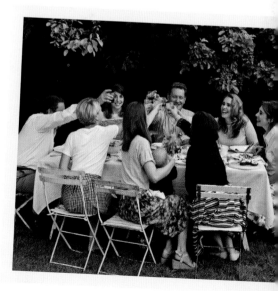

BABY, TODDLER, FAMILY

With the ultimate aim of making your favourite meals their favourite flavours, the book is structured into three sections, from first weaning steps to picky-toddler snacks to your baby eating the same meal as you at the table. It is divided into three sections: Baby (weaning), Toddler (snacks) and Family (one meal).

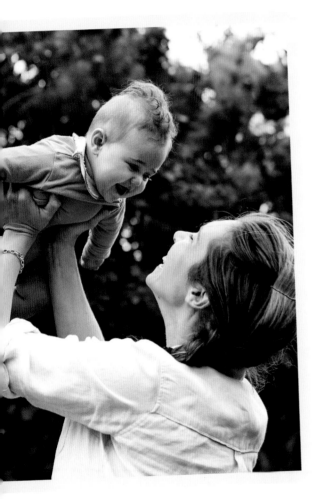

BABY: WEANING

Start them young.
We believe food should be at the heart of every child's upbringing and that it should start as early as possible. So, starting right from the weaning stages, this book shares our tips and experiences for any parent keen to encourage their child to appreciate good wholesome food. Weaning forms the building blocks of raising a child to enjoy food for life.

ABC Weaning Steps.
There is so much information available (often contradictory) that it can be really confusing for new parents. I was overwhelmed when I started weaning my baby, and Emi was faced with exactly the same dilemma when it was her turn. So, with the help of nutritionists, both from Italy and the UK, we have cherry-picked the best advice and produced our simple guide to baby weaning the Italian way. By the age of 1 your baby should be eating meals with the whole family, with maybe only a small tweak here and there with regard to seasonings and certain ingredients.

The 'Baby' section of the book talks you through the ABC Weaning Steps – tips, tricks and what to avoid.

A: INTRODUCING FLAVOURS (6-8 MONTHS)

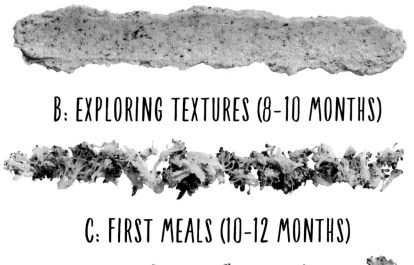

B: EXPLORING TEXTURES (8-10 MONTHS)

C: FIRST MEALS (10-12 MONTHS)

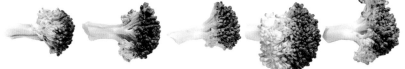

Simplicity.

When we started weaning, we looked for tips and recipes online, but so many ideas went down the plughole because they were completely impractical for a busy mum. Either they had too many ingredients (which went to waste), or they involved too many pots and pans. No one wants to make a purée the size of a walnut with an hour of washing-up afterwards!

Our ABC recipes are all about practicality.

♦ **Baby Brodino** (see page 68) for first tastes

♦ **No-cook purées** that can be whizzed up in seconds, meaning you can avoid reaching for the emergency supermarket pouch!

♦ **Pick 'n' Mix Cubes** for when you're out and about (see page 74)

♦ **Textured meals and finger foods** to help your baby progress to first meals

TODDLER: SNACKS

Daytime fixes.
During the day, family schedules can often be jam-packed and out of sync, so Emi and I created this section of the book to give recipes that are great for snacks, lunchboxes, play-dates and speedy meals.

Toddler challenges and picky eaters.
Before writing this book, I spoke with a huge number of mums, asking them what challenges they faced when it came to mealtimes and their kids. There were lots of similar voices here…

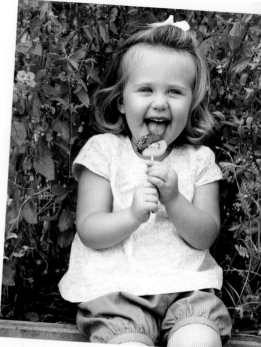

♦ '**Packed lunches** are always a struggle – how do I give variety without the stress?'

♦ '**I'm always running late** and often need a quick lunch solution for my hungry toddler, which means the old faithful cheese-and-ham sarnies continuously get wheeled out…How do I mix things up with only 5 minutes' preparation time?'

♦ '**It's always a struggle** thinking of simple breakfast ideas…so I just go for the easy option and hand over the cereal box.'

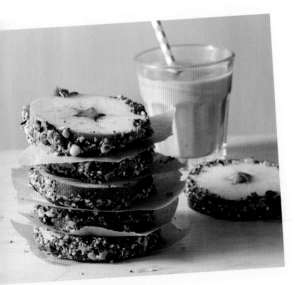

WE HAVE ANSWERED SOME OF THESE CHALLENGES IN THE TODDLER RECIPE SECTION (SEE PAGES 114–61).

FAMILY: ONE MEAL

One family. One meal.

If you follow our easy 3-step plan, by the age of 1 your baby should be able to eat a version of the same meal you feed the rest of the family. All the recipes in this section are practical, simple, quick and nutritious for a busy parent, and they include plenty of variations, so that you can adapt the same meal for a baby, toddler or adult.

15 minutes' prep time.

We know how hard it can be for parents to juggle busy lives, but we don't think your cooking should suffer as a consequence. Emi and I have shared our tips and recipes for how everyone can cook fresh, easy and delicious meals at any time of day. You might need to let some recipes simmer, stew or brew for longer, but for the majority, the time you have to dedicate to the kitchen stove should be less than 15 minutes.

This section includes:

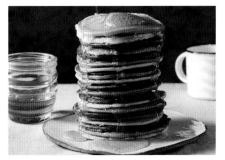

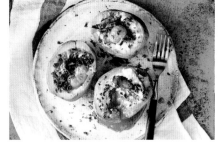

BRUNCHES (page175)

SPEEDY DINNERS (page186)

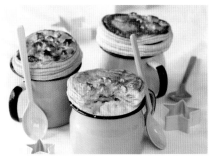

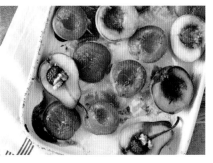

ONE-POT MEALS
(page 211)

DESSERTS AND BAKES
(page 236)

A FEW THINGS
ABOUT THIS BOOK

We know how precious kids' sleep time can be ... if you're lucky you might have 45 minutes to yourself while the baby naps and over a hundred chores to get done, when all you want is to put your feet up on the sofa and have forty winks! That's why recipes with a quick preparation time are key.

Minimal ingredients.

We have tried to keep our ingredients lists to an absolute minimum. The last thing you want is a recipe that requires you to buy the entire contents of the supermarket and leaves you with lots of random leftover ingredients at the end. Where possible, we've stripped back recipes to keep the ingredients to a minimum and the methods nice and simple.

Store-cupboard essentials.

A well-stocked store cupboard and freezer will make your life so much easier. See page 22 for our Get Ahead Essentials list. Then, when it comes to cooking, you need only shop for a few 'To buy' ingredients. For some recipes, you might not even need to go shopping at all.

Minimum preparation time and washing up.

We binned recipes that involved too many steps or complicated methods.

Cheeky twists on classics.

The recipes in this book are all about giving you simple solutions, so we challenged the methods of many traditional recipes and turned them on their head. Check out the Beef Bolognese on page 217, which has a preparation time of 15 minutes and is packed with loads of hidden veggies. The results are just as tasty as the traditional method, but it means you can juggle ten other errands at the same time. Home-cooked food does not have to be put on the back burner when you're busy!

A blob of this. A splash of that.

When pushed for time, we always avoid recipes that have fiddly measurements or lots of careful weighing. We know that when it comes to baking, precise measurements are important, but in most day-to-day cooking that's not required. We're big believers in simplicity and in the idea that flavours should drive the measures ... Our nonna (grandmother), like most Italian cooks, never weighed a thing! It should be about TASTE, TASTE, TASTE, not specific instructions. That's why, in this book, you'll see that lots of measurements are kept simple.

Plenty of choice and flexibility.

Where possible, we've tried to give lots of flexibility and options in the recipes. For example, if you haven't got butternut squash, try using sweet potatoes or carrots. We want you to get excited about the alternatives you can create. Feeding a family is about providing lots of variety, and you should have the confidence to mix things up and try the same dish ten different ways.

Gluten free (G), Dairy free (D), Free from added sugar (S), Vegetarian (V).

More and more people are following a particular diet or finding themselves intolerant of certain food groups, so we have included some recipes that they can enjoy too. Ironically, some of our favourite recipes are naturally vegetarian, gluten free or free from added sugar, but if labelled that way it's possible that the average person won't give them a go. So for this reason, we have listed whether recipes are G, D, S or V in the index only.

Nutrition health check.

All the recipes in this book have been checked by an approved nutritionist to verify that they comply with national food standards.

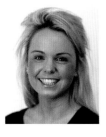

Meet the expert.

All the advice in this book has been approved by Rozzie Batchelar, who graduated from Oxford Brookes University with a BSc in Nutrition and Sports and Exercise Science, and has been a registered food nutritionist with the Association for Nutrition since 2012. She has been working for the Jamie Oliver Media Group for four years and works across all areas of food nutrition, most notably recipe analysis, nutrition and health claims, recipe development, sports nutrition, infant nutrition and complementary feeding and nutrition for special diets.

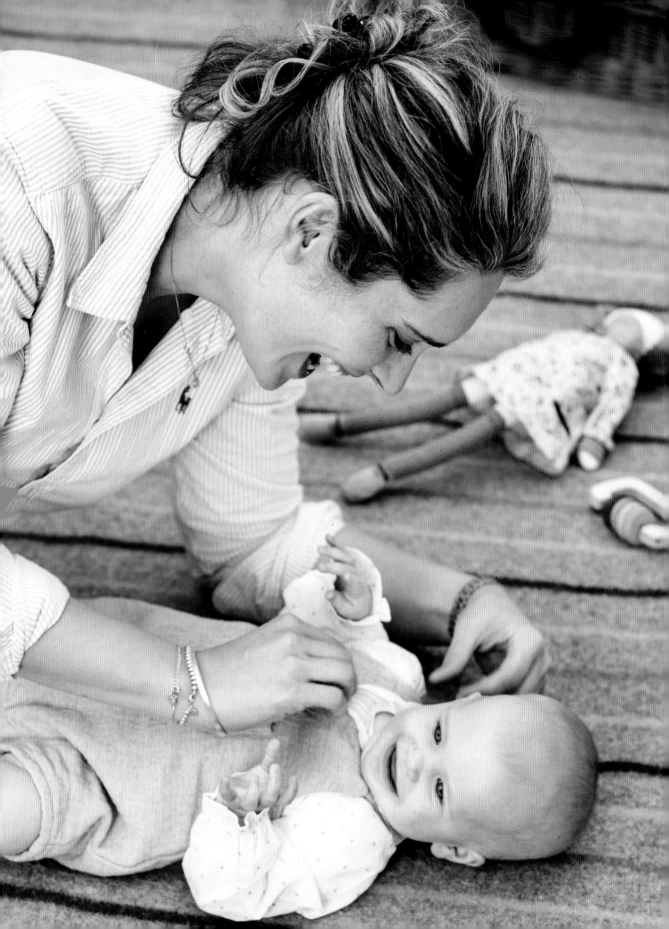

GET AHEAD ESSENTIALS

In the following pages, we have listed those absolute essentials that you might not currently have, which will form the backbone of your family cooking and make the experience a breeze. If we can give you only one piece of advice before you start your weaning journey, it's to do the following three things:

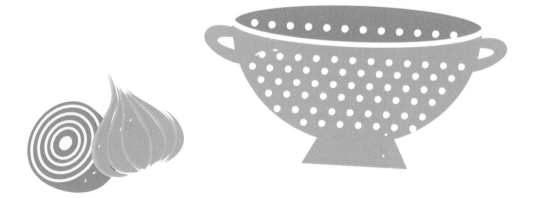

1
**ORGANIZE
YOUR FREEZER**

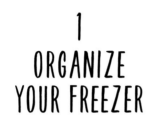

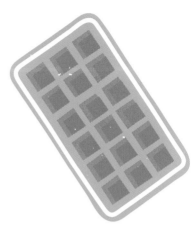

2
**BUY YOUR
BASIC EQUIPMENT**

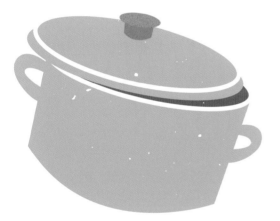

3
**STOCK UP YOUR
STORE CUPBOARD**

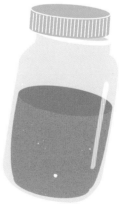

THE ESSENTIALS: YOUR FREEZER

The freezer is your power source for becoming a whiz in the kitchen ... Learning how to use it efficiently will turn you into Super-Mum!

Try answering these questions first:

Can you list everything that is in your freezer without opening the door?

Are there things in your freezer that have been there longer than 3 months?

If you've forgotten what's in your freezer or things have been sitting there for months (if not years!), it's definitely time to get sorted! Here are my tips for helping you get your freezer organized:

CLEAR IT OUT

You won't believe how refreshing it can be to start again with an empty freezer. Your freezer will become your holy grail, and to use it properly you need space and order. Spend a week (or two) using up the contents of the freezer before you start getting organized. Check there is no build-up of ice - if your freezer has chunks of ice growing from the sides, you need to defrost it before you start. You can gain lots of extra space by getting rid of the ice build-up.

SPACE

Always make sure you rotate and use your freezer 'meals' regularly and have space to spare. That way you can easily see what's in the freezer and also have room for storing good leftovers.

STORAGE:

A good-quality ice-cube tray. Ideally a silicone one as it's easier to clean and pop the cubes out.

Freezer bags. These are the best way to store food, as they use minimal space. You can also use them to store liquids/soups - just freeze them flat so they are easier to stack. Buy a selection of sizes, make sure they are well sealed and try to remove any air pockets before you close them.

Disposable foil containers. These are absolutely brilliant for freezing individually portioned meals such as lasagna, casseroles, etc., and putting them straight into the oven from frozen - your own home-cooked ready meals. We get quite possessive about these meals, as they are life-savers in an emergency, so we save them for moments of desperation! Get containers that are all the same size so they are easier to stack (small rectangular ones are best). Note that when cooking from frozen, you should always check that the food is fully cooked through.

LABEL EVERYTHING

Keep a permanent black marker in your cutlery drawer. Label everything that goes into your freezer with the recipe/ingredients and the date it went in. (We have been known to use frozen kale instead of parsley because we forgot to label the bag!)

YOUR FREEZER SUPPLIES

I cannot emphasize strongly enough how vital your freezer will be in helping you make the best meals for your family in record time. The following are supplies we always keep in the freezer and that are essential for emergency meals. If you ever start to run low on any of these, make sure you get them put on your shopping list and stocked up ASAP, as you never want to be without.

Find a spare hour at the weekend to prepare your freezer supplies – it will save you oodles of time when preparing emergency mid-week meals!

KALE CRUMBS

Everyone harps on about how great the superfood kale is, but I have to be honest – I find it a really tough and bitter leaf to digest. No wonder kids turn their noses up at it! Solution – buy a bag of kale and immediately blitz it (without cooking it), until it forms a fine powder. Then bag it up and put it into the freezer. You can scoop it out when you need it and throw it into anything you fancy – soups, omelettes, stews, even pancakes. It's so fine that the kids don't even notice it and yet they are getting all the goodness!

HERBS

Herbs are brilliant for seasoning, especially for babies, who can't have added salt. But how many of you have bought a basil or parsley plant that has turned limp before you've had time to use it? Solution – the best way to store your herbs is in the freezer, and they defrost in seconds. You can throw them straight into your meals!

Finely chop rosemary, parsley, basil or mint (or blitz with a stick blender) and bag them up for the freezer, ready to use whenever you fancy (remember to label them!).

You can also put your chopped or blitzed herbs into ice-cube trays and pour over olive oil to make them into herby cubes. Once frozen, pop the cubes into a freezer bag to minimize storage and free up the ice-cube tray for using again. Great as a base for many soups, stews, etc.

GRATED PARMESAN

We can't live without a bag of grated Parmesan in the fridge – the bigger, the better! We always buy Parmesan fresh (as a block, and never in ready-grated tubs), but we grate it straight away and then bag it up for the freezer – yes, it requires elbow grease, but it saves you a trip to the gym. It stays at its freshest this way and you can just grab it by the handful when you need it. You might think it's expensive, but it's a brilliant form of seasoning that means you use less salt.

BREADCRUMBS

Just slice your bread or use any old bits of crust. Put them into a bowl and leave them to air-dry for a few days. Don't use processed supermarket sliced bread, as this tends to go mouldy before it dries out. Baguettes or loaves from a good bakery are best. Once the bread is rock hard, put it into your blender in batches and blitz it to fine crumbs. Put it into a freezer bag (label it) and it's all done! The bigger the bag of crumbs the better, and keep it regularly stocked up.

Ryvita crackers are also great for making crumbs if you are struggling to build up your stale bread supply.

FROZEN VEG

Always keep some frozen veg in your freezer that cooks super-fast (I keep a bag of peas and one of leaf spinach).

FROZEN MEAT AND FISH

Frozen fish fillets. (We like cod and salmon.) These are often on offer from the supermarket and are much cheaper than buying fresh. It means you always have a speedy protein meal if you forget to go to the shops.

Frozen chicken fillets. (We like to keep about 6 fillets at a time in the freezer in case of unexpected guests.) Freeze them in individual bags so they are quicker to defrost and you can pull out only the number you need.

FROZEN FRUIT

Frozen berries. Cheaper than buying fresh, and brilliant for giving kids some great afternoon treats.

Frozen bananas. Everyone has one or two bananas in the bunch that go a little too squidgy and brown to enjoy fresh. Peel them, cut them in half and put them into a freezer bag. Frozen bananas are fantastic for making a super-quick gelato treat for the kids (see page 160).

Smoothie bags. Take a little time to prepare some smoothie bags. Cut up a range of your favourite fruits and divide them between small freezer bags (e.g a kiwi, some berries, a few pieces of mango and half a banana). This provides you with a 1-minute snack or smoothie any time of day (see page140–41).

THE ESSENTIALS: YOUR EQUIPMENT

Cookery books often include a long list of equipment but I'm going to do the opposite. I'm going to assume most of you already have a sharp knife, a chopping board, a saucepan/frying pan and a sieve.

Here are the absolute essentials; the equipment you really must have to make your life easier in the kitchen.

A LARGE HEAVY-BASED SAUCEPAN

with a lid that can cook a risotto, boil water for pasta, simmer a stew and brown meat.

A SPEED PEELER

(NOT a knife peeler)

FOIL, CLINGFILM, BAKING PAPER

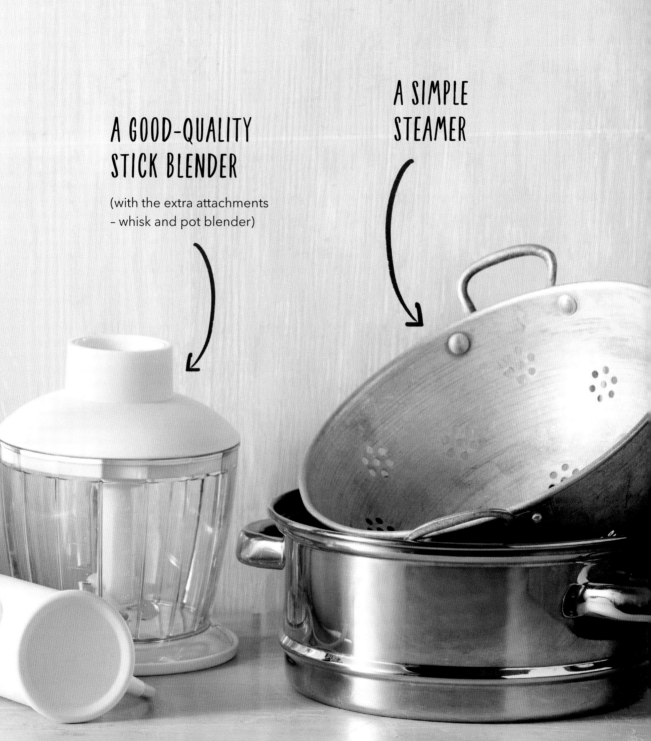

A GOOD-QUALITY STICK BLENDER

(with the extra attachments – whisk and pot blender)

A SIMPLE STEAMER

FREEZER EQUIPMENT

(ice-cube trays, foil trays, bags, containers – see page 25)

THE ESSENTIALS: YOUR STORE CUPBOARD

All the recipes in this book have the ingredients list divided into two sections: the 'To buy' ingredients and the 'Store-cupboard essentials'. If you can always be sure to have the following ingredients in your store cupboard, it will make your cooking life so much easier. Get into the habit of doubling up on these items – that way you can keep them ticking over and never run out.

In every Italian kitchen . . .
Onions and garlic
Tinned tomatoes
Olive oil and extra virgin olive oil
Parmesan cheese

Fillers
2 packets of pasta
2 packets of pastina
1 packet of basmati rice
1 packet of Arborio rice
Oats

Dairy
Eggs
Milk
Butter

Fish
2–3 tins of tuna, salmon or
sardines in spring water or oil.
**Avoid ones in brine and with
added salt.**

Dried fruit and nuts
A selection of dried fruits
and nuts (cashews, hazelnuts,
pecans etc.).

Herbs and spices
Ground ginger
Ground cinnamon
Dried rosemary
Dried oregano
Salt and pepper

Legumes
2–3 tins of beans (cannellini,
borlotti, chickpeas, lentils, etc.)
**without added salt, sugar or
sodium additive. This will be
very clearly labelled.**

Baking
Plain flour
Self-raising flour
Caster sugar
Honey and/or pure maple syrup
Vanilla extract
Bicarbonate of soda
Baking powder

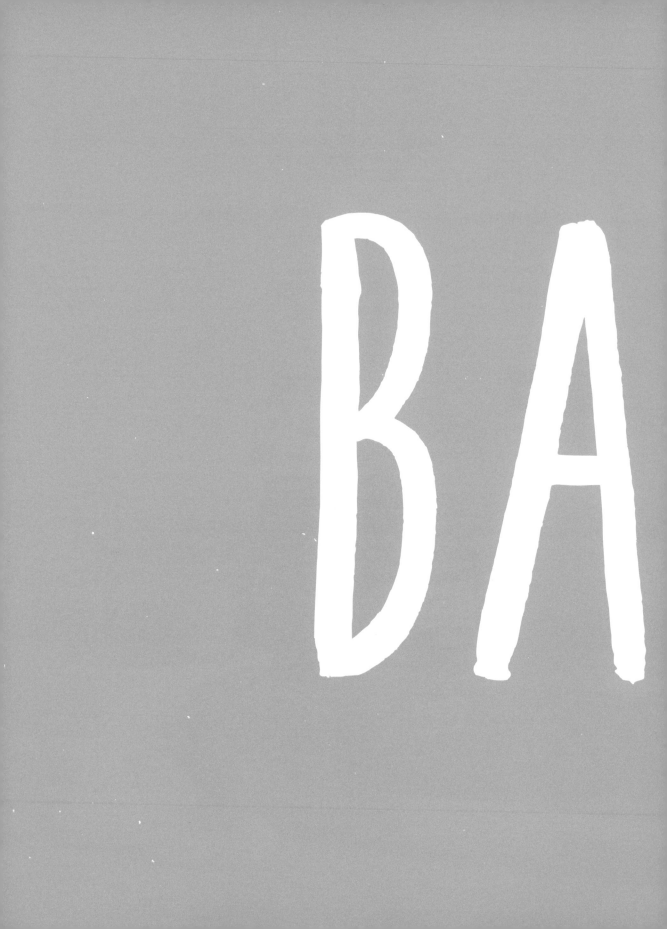

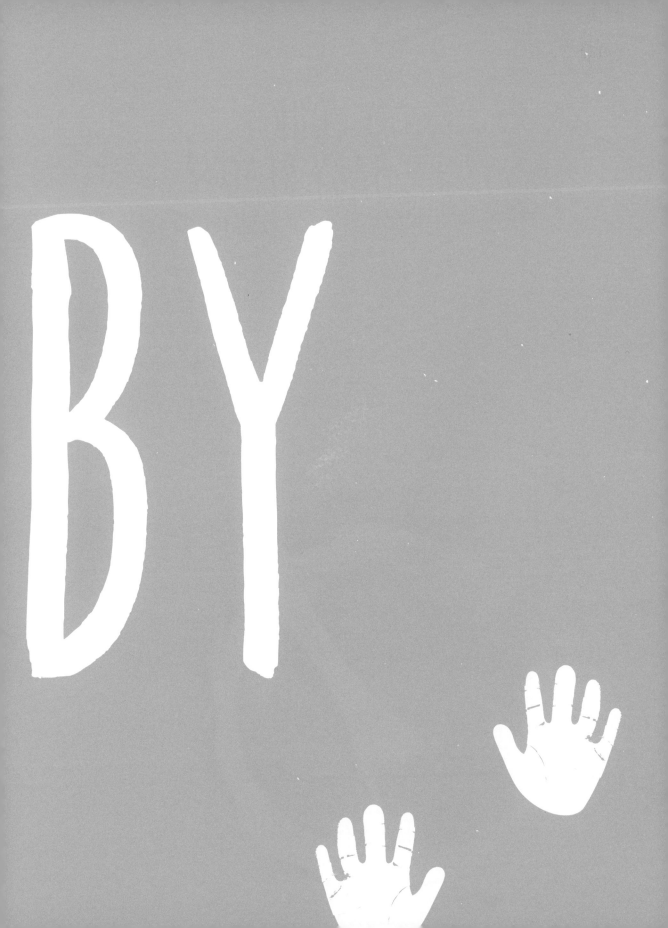

IS YOUR BABY READY?

When to start weaning?

There are lots of opinions about when a baby is ready to start weaning. Some parents mistake the signs and wean too early – common myths about babies being ready are chewing their fingers/hands/fists, grabbing other people's food, demanding more milk, sleepless nights, or waking up when they have been sleeping through. These are not necessarily signs of a baby wanting more food! The bottom line is to try to wait until your baby is as close to 6 months as possible.

Why wait until 6 months?

♦ By 6 months, a baby's digestive system is more fully formed, which will help them digest a wider range of foods. They will also have developed the ability to swallow at this point.

♦ Any sooner and you may find you have to stick to baby rice and bland basic vegetable purées. As a result your baby may get too dependent on these and start turning their nose up at more interesting flavours and textures later on (which can be the start of fussy-eater problems).

♦ By 6 months your baby can eat almost anything (there are only a few foods to avoid – see page 40). So there is less stress for you and it's more fun and exciting for the baby.

♦ By 6 months a baby can usually sit up straighter, holding their head upright, making it easier for them to digest food and running less of a risk of choking.

♦ By 6 months your baby should have developed a natural reflex to push food to the back of their mouth to swallow (apparently, if they look like they're licking their lips it's actually them learning to push food around in their mouth and not necessarily a sign they're saying, 'Mmmm, that was tasty!'). However, it is also possible for babies to lose this reflex if you have not started to introduce food by the 6-month mark. So while it is important to wait until your baby is ready, it's also crucial not to delay weaning too much past the 6-month mark.

What are the signs to look for?

♦ A baby should be able to sit up comfortably (almost without support or unaided) and hold their head up.

♦ Good head control is key, as it means the baby will have good muscular coordination, which will allow them to learn to swallow food easily.

♦ A baby should be able to reach out and grasp food and put it up to their mouth.

What's the official line?

The WHO (World Health Organization) advises exclusive milk feeding until 6 months.

Some exceptions such as premature babies might need to be weaned earlier. But a GP will be the best person to advise this.

Every baby is individual, though, and there's no one-size-fits-all. Check if your baby is showing the developmental signs mentioned on the previous page. Be guided by your baby and your health visitor or GP.

Never wean before 17 weeks, as the baby's organs are not developed enough to process foods. Before 4 months, a baby is physiologically unable to digest food.

By 6 months, your baby can eat just about anything

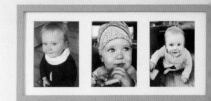

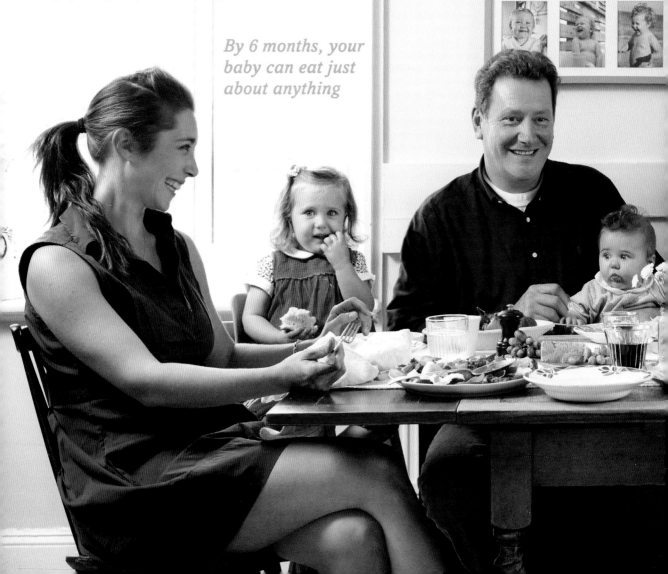

What worked for me.

So, when to start weaning? Well, as you can imagine I've had MASSIVE pressure from everyone in my Italian family about weaning – everyone has had an opinion (even my dad!). Ever since Fiamma was born, my father was obsessed with wanting to put food into her mouth. Every day he would ask, 'Can I give her some coffee yet?', 'What about some vino?', 'How about some milk? Cream? Cheese?' No, Dad!

I decided to follow the advice of my health visitor and the medical standards, which highlight huge benefits in waiting as close to 6 months as possible. I started weaning Fiamma a week before she turned 6 months and she took to it brilliantly. We were able to give her a huge variety of foods in a short space of time, which I believe helped her enjoy her meals.

WHAT TO AVOID

There are lots of opinions about what you should avoid for your baby and I found the variations quite overwhelming! In the end, I took the advice of a number of health professionals both in the UK and in Italy, who said that at 6 months your baby can eat most foods – there is just a small list of those to avoid. The only things to be cautious of to start with are allergens (gluten, eggs, milk, fish and peanuts, for example). Once your baby is 6 months, feel free to explore foods from all the different food groups. This is what my grandmother would have done years ago, so why obsess about it now? Less to worry about, more fun!

The one thing that I would stress here, though, is that processed foods are as bad as junk fast foods. If you choose not to take your kids to McDonald's, then don't let them eat sugary breakfast cereals, processed sauces or ready meals either.

The following are the only absolute no-nos recommended by health practitioners.

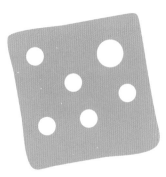

Honey. With honey there is a small risk of a food-poisoning bacterium that can cause infant botulism, so it's recommended that you avoid it until your baby is 1 year old.

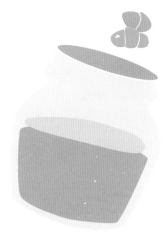

Unpasteurized foods and blue cheeses. I gave Fiamma Brie, Gorgonzola and other cheeses just as they do in Italy, so use your judgement.

Shark, marlin, swordfish and liver. These may contain heavy metals or pollutants, or too much of one vitamin.

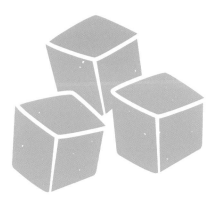

Sugar and artificial sweeteners. They're not needed and you don't want your baby to get too used to sweet foods; very few kids say no to sweet treats and it's better to get them hooked on savoury first. High amounts of sugar can also cause tooth decay. Again, no need to panic if your baby dips her fingers in the sugar bowl or has a cheeky taste of some chocolate; but best to avoid this where possible. Steer clear of ultra-sweet foods that can damage teeth and try to give fruit as part of a meal.

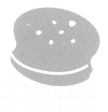

Salt. It's not needed for children under 2 years, and can overload your baby's developing kidneys. Also, keep salty foods (e.g. bacon, cured meats, smoked fish, olives and brine-preserved foods) to a minimum until your baby is at least 1 year old. There is no harm in letting your baby try these foods (great for variety and new tastes); however, it should really be for a taste only rather than for nutrition.

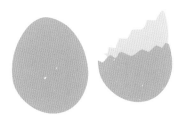

Raw shellfish and uncooked eggs. This is because of the risk of food poisoning; however, use your judgement again here. We are all at risk of food poisoning when eating raw eggs, but Italians live on desserts such as tiramisu. If you buy good-quality produce and are confident about what you are eating, feel free to let your little one have a taste – I did. I think it's wonderful to allow them to explore lots of flavours.

Before 6 months: If you choose to introduce food before 6 months, you should exclude wheat and gluten in cereal foods such as bread and pasta, eggs, nuts and seeds, liver, fish, shellfish and cows' milk or other dairy foods. Basically stick to simple and starchy vegetables (such as potatoes, carrots, courgettes) and baby rice.

And here are a few extra things nutritionists advise against:

Low-fat foods and diet 'sugar-free' drinks. Avoid these if possible, as they are full of sugar or unnatural preservatives and sweeteners, which can be really bad for your health. Exceptions can be made in the case of some low-fat natural yoghurts or Greek yoghurts, and semi-skimmed and skimmed milks are free from nasties and added sugar. However, babies should ALWAYS be eating full-fat versions of foods, as they need the energy. Note: rice milk should never be given to babies or children under 5, as it contains arsenic in amounts that may be dangerous for small children.

Fizzy drinks, squashes, cordials and fruit juices. These are high in unnecessary sugars that no one needs; not adults, not toddlers, and certainly not your baby. They also encourage a sweet tooth and can cause tooth decay. And yes, I include natural fruit juices in this list. It's better for you to eat a whole orange than it is to drink the juice (which is essentially just sugar and has had the fibre stripped out of it).

Caffeine and alcohol. Avoid any drinks that have tannins or caffeine in them, and drinks that contain acid or alcohol. Equally, don't get paranoid if your kid tries a cake with liqueur in it or if they dip a finger in your coffee (our kids have had a try of both at some point – unavoidable in an Italian home) – I believe it's about common sense.

Processed foods or sauces, and foods containing artificial food colouring. Most breakfast cereals, ketchup, processed pasta sauces, processed cakes and biscuits, crisps and ready meals are FULL of salt, sugar and other artificial additives and ingredients. Much better to give your family a speedy home-cooked meal than fill them with processed foods (which in my opinion can be just as bad as junk fast food!).

Brown or wholegrain foods. Great for adults, but for babies these higher-fibre foods mean they may get full before they have got all the nutrients and energy they need. Wholegrains should be consumed in small quantities by babies and infants, and a combination of white and wholemeal is best for them.

Foods that can cause choking. These include whole nuts, whole grapes and, for babies, chunks of hard foods such as apple or cheese.

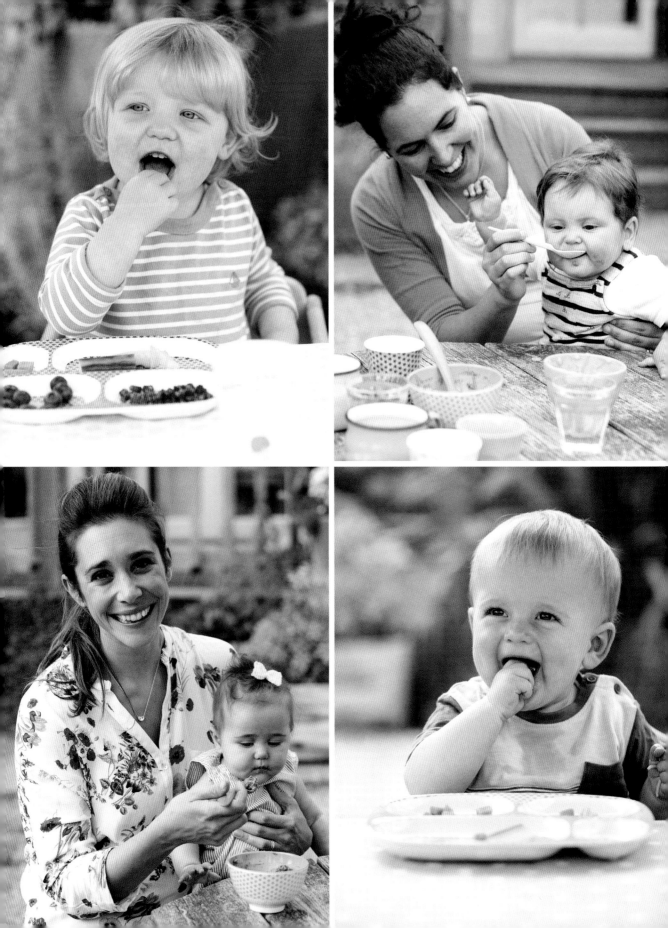

WEANING: HOW MUCH FOOD TO GIVE?

When I started weaning, I really struggled with understanding quantities. Lots of people say your baby will tell you when they are full . . . Ha! Not mine . . . she had no off button!

So what to do? My nonna and my mum told me to think about something visual (a tablespoon, her fist size, a yoghurt pot) and take the measurements from there.

The current nutritional advice (source: www.firststepsnutrition.org) is:

6 MONTHS

A baby's tummy is very small (see opposite page), and the best solution is to start by giving 2-3 teaspoons, and every now and again just up the quantity.

7-9 MONTHS

From this age your baby will probably have about 250 calories a day from food but, like adults, their appetites will vary from meal to meal and day to day, and it is important to trust your baby. Keep offering a range of foods at meals; let the baby be an active eater and offer milk feeds morning and night and before naps if this pattern works well. Use the responsive feeding cues learnt in the first 6 months to follow your baby's lead.

10-12 MONTHS

From this age your baby will be getting about 450 calories a day from food, split up into approximately 3 meals. Babies will regulate their milk intake as they eat more food, and remember that each day may be different in terms of how much food and milk the baby has.

Here you can see just how small a baby's tummy can be:

Day 1
Size of a hazelnut

One week
Size of a kiwi

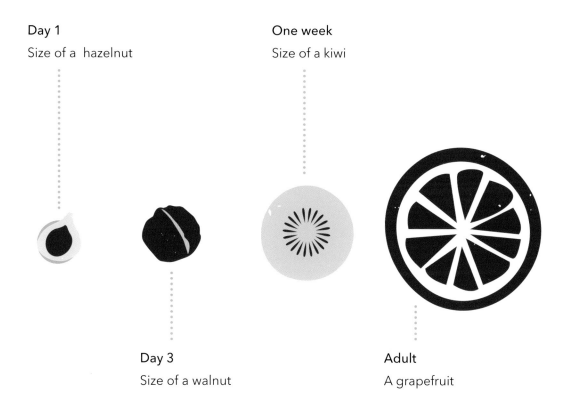

Day 3
Size of a walnut

Adult
A grapefruit

What worked for me

When I started weaning Fiamma, I began by visualizing large tablespoon sizes but quickly increased this to about 3-4 tablespoons, letting her guide me.

By about 8 months, she was eating about the equivalent of 2 or 3 of her fists (not your fist . . . the baby's fist!).

This shouldn't be stressful – let your baby be your guide, and don't forget that they are also getting a large quantity of nutrients from your breast milk or formula.

HOW MUCH FOOD?

	FOOD	NUTRITION
0-6 MONTHS	Up to 6 months, exclusively milk (formula and/or breast milk).	**milk = nutrition** Breast milk or formula dominates your baby's diet for the first year, and this is where they will get most of their nutrients and vitamins.
6-8 MONTHS	Breast milk or formula is still the main source of nutrition. Approximate food quantities: 1-2 teaspoons or a few mouthfuls of food at the start of the weaning process. Increase to approx. 2-3 tablespoons per meal.	**milk = nutrition** **food = variety** Iron is one of the nutrients that starts to run low as your baby grows, so plenty of greens are a good way to boost iron levels and vitamin c.
8-12 MONTHS	The balance starts to shift - food provides additional nutrients (see pages 257–59) but breast milk or formula are still a vital source of nutrition too.	**milk = nutrition** **food = nutrition & variety** A baby's food intake should start to increase along with different textures and flavours. A baby will still require breast milk or formula but this will slowly start to reduce naturally.

TEXTURE

WATER

Cooled boiled water or filtered tap water is ok. Avoid mineral water, as most of these contain high salt levels or added minerals.

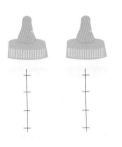

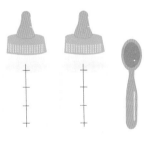

Food is about learning new flavours and textures. Variety is key. By 8 months baby could be having 3 'meals' a day of approximately 1–2 portions of her fist size.

Filtered tap water can be given with meals. If baby goes off milk when introduced to food, add their milk (breast/formula) to your cooking to continue giving them the nutrients.

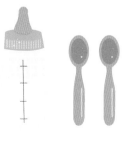

Variety, flavours and textures are also very important – if you are still feeding purées, try to move quickly on to more textures and chunkier foods.

More meals means your baby requires more fluid. Introduce lidded beakers and sippy cups instead of bottles with teats. Try giving your baby a drink from an open cup too.

WEANING: WHAT MEAL DO I START WITH?

When I began introducing food, I had to decide which meal to start with. Pick the meal that is the easiest for you!

Weaning is a new experience and a challenge, especially if you are a busy person, so make it as easy as possible for you to manage. It's also important to be as consistent as possible in the early weeks, giving the baby clear signs of when they can expect their mealtime.

For me, breakfast was the easiest meal by far – we were always home and it was the one I could be most consistent with. Lunchtime was the hardest, as we were often out and about.

It's also very important not to drop any of your breastfeeds/milk feeds when you start weaning. At 6 months your baby is still getting all the nutrients they need from milk, and weaning is more about getting her used to new flavours and textures quickly than it is about giving extra nutrients. I would always give a 'meal' or solids after a breastfeed rather than before – you need your baby to be on good form, not ravenous, as you want her to develop a positive relationship with food.

What to feed your baby for the first time.
Our nonna always said it's a really good plan to keep breakfast as simple and consistent as possible, for a number of reasons:

(a) The last thing you want to do is have the stress of being creative with your cooking when you've had a sleepless night. You need something you can do on autopilot at 6 a.m. There is plenty of time to experiment with flavours and textures for lunch and dinner.

(b) Simplicity and routine in the morning means you are in a calm (or calmer) state of mind, and it should also mean you don't start your day with endless washing up after an attempt at a new recipe goes wrong.

(c) Being consistent with one meal of the day is a really helpful indicator of whether your baby is ill/teething/out of sorts. If my baby rejected any meals, I would try to make excuses or find it hard to work out whether it was her starting to get fussy or whether it was too hot/too cold/not a nice flavour or texture, etc. However, being at least consistent with breakfast means that if the baby rejects it after weeks of enjoying it, that should be an easy indicator that something is not quite right (teething/cold, etc.). And a baby can reject a food up to 10 times before accepting it, so it's worth persevering with new foods every so often after an initial rejection, rather than giving up on the food altogether.

What worked for me

So we started with baby porridge or baby rice with some of my breast milk (you can also use formula). I felt it was the most natural thing to start with, as using milk to mix the porridge/rice helped her identify flavours she was already used to.

After a few days I started to introduce an evening 'meal'. This is where I began Step A of my baby weaning plan (see page 45), and Baby Brodino (see page 68) was the most simple way to start. After another few days I started to mix up my Baby Brodino by using different veg and adding a spoonful of olive oil and a sprinkling of Parmesan.

After a couple of weeks, I changed the texture of the Baby Brodino from a loose and smooth consistency to a thicker/lumpier texture. I then started introducing first foods, following the ABC Weaning Steps (see page 58).

By 8 months my baby had tasted all the main food groups and was also eating a mixture of textures and finger foods. It's always good to have finger food available even if you are feeding the baby yourself from a spoon, as it encourages baby-led feeding, i.e. it gets babies learning how to pick up food and feed themselves!

SEE PAGE 181
FOR PORRIDGE RECIPES

BABY-LED WEANING

OK, so I'm probably going to start quite a debate here, but I want to give you my family's opinion on baby-led weaning. I have spoken to my mum, my Italian family and my great-aunts a lot about it, and I was really curious about its theory – letting children take the lead to encourage them to take control and be confident with food (i.e. to prevent them becoming fussy eaters and having problems when they become toddlers). Ultimately I am trying to achieve the same goal, but somehow I found the process of letting a baby be FULLY in control a little strange.

My instinct as a mum is to ensure my baby is getting the right nutrients and food for her growth. Well, whenever I gave Fiamma any finger food, I was never 100 per cent certain how much she had actually swallowed. Had she actually eaten all that banana or had half of it got squished in her top, under her bum, mashed in the rug or flung on the opposite wall?

My sisters and I were brought up loving our food and mealtimes; however, we were taught 'old-school' style with a spoon. Why do it any differently?

However, the concept of giving babies finger food is a good one – it has certainly let Fiamma understand how to take sensible bites and not choke, and it's a fantastic support if you have a hungry baby on your hands but dinner's not quite ready. A stick of pepper or a slice of apple keeps them entertained in moments of panic!

However, I don't believe this should be the primary method of feeding; I tend to give some finger foods before or after the 'meal'. I want my children to grow up eating like kids do on the continent – eating meals politely with the adults, eating a variety of foods and certainly not using mealtimes as a time to play with food.

And I don't let Fiamma shovel porridge, pasta or anything similar with her hands – I'm old school too, and I do believe children understand discipline from an early age and do not need to dive head first into bowls of mashed potato. Of course, it's hard for a toddler to eat spaghetti neatly, and sometimes the job's too big for a bib!

THE ABC OF WEANING

I've developed this plan to help parents cook fresh and healthy food while keeping things easy. Three simple steps to give you a basic guide with plenty of flexibility. By the end of the ABC Weaning Steps, your baby should be ready to eat a version of your family meal.

Each step should take approximately 2 months, so by the time your baby is 1, weaning should be complete. Simple!

Weaning your baby is less about nutrition in the early stages and MUCH MORE ABOUT VARIETY – this is so important. Your baby needs to experience as many different flavours and textures as possible, and giving lots of diversity will help prevent them becoming fussy eaters in the future. So the more you can mix things up, the better!

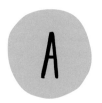 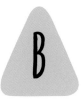 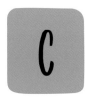

Step A:
INTRODUCING
FLAVOURS
6–8 months

Step B:
EXPLORING
TEXTURES
8–10 months

Step C:
FIRST MEALS
10–12 months

A

INTRODUCING FLAVOURS
6-8 MONTHS

This is all about first tastes. Put simply, a baby can eat almost anything by 6 months. There are very few things a baby cannot eat, and these are listed on page 40 (you mainly need to avoid salt and sugar, honey, unpasteurized foods and raw fish/meat/eggs).

It's good to introduce the main food groups one by one, to help ease in your baby's digestive system and also check for allergies. Try to get through these introductions as quickly as possible, otherwise spending too long on one food group will risk your baby getting used to one thing and possibly becoming a picky eater. Babies are OK eating from all the different food groups from 6 months. However, here is the order I went for. Vegetables are always a great starting point.

1. **Vegetables and fruits**

2. **Meats and eggs** (first white meats and fish, then red meats)

3. **Gluten, nuts and pulses**

B

EXPLORING TEXTURES
8-10 MONTHS

As soon as the first foods have been introduced, you can begin to have fun and start introducing new flavours and textures. Don't delay this stage, as a baby who has only had runny purées until 9 months can completely reject lumps and make mealtimes a real challenge. Moving quickly through different textures will help your baby learn how to bite and chew safely, and will also help with speech development. It's always daunting to give your baby new textures, for fear of choking (especially if they don't have many, or any, teeth). However, if you introduce them slowly and observe their progress the whole time, you'll be amazed how your little one will learn how to chew and move the new textures around in their mouth. One meal a day really should contain meat or fish, as by 8 months a baby needs the additional nutrients they provide (protein, vitamin B, zinc, iron and omega 3 fatty acids). Note that vegetarians can get these nutrients from eggs, dairy, green leafy veg, nuts and seeds. This is where you can really start to experiment with textures and flavours, such as herbs and spices, different cheeses, pasta shapes and lots of new finger foods. Start mashing cooked purées with a fork where possible, or add pastina shapes – start with soft lumps and then move on to harder textures.

C

FIRST MEALS
10-12 MONTHS

Once your baby is used to lots of different flavours and textures you should start getting them used to having 3 meals a day, and whole meals. It's time to start cooking meals that the whole family can enjoy. By now your baby should be really used to eating more lumps, textures and harder finger foods. Milk should still be a main part of their diet (either formula or breast milk), but they can now eat energy-rich solid foods too.

Added salt and sugar should still be kept out of the baby's diet, and honey and processed foods should also be avoided. Try to encourage the use of a beaker or cup for drinking water, and the development of the pincer grip with lots of finger foods.

STEP A: INTRODUCING FIRST FOODS

This is probably the most important stage of weaning. By introducing the main food groups step by step, you can keep an eye out for potential allergies but also let your baby get used to different flavours and textures slowly.

The best advice I was given was not to overthink this stage. As a general rule, babies can eat almost any foods from 6 months, so don't get too stressed out about what they can and can't have. Try to have fun! It's really important that you wait until your baby is 6 months before you start weaning. Before 6 months your baby's digestive system isn't fully formed, so the foods you can give are much more limited. A variety of flavours and textures is much more important than quantity at this stage, so don't be afraid if your baby rejects a meal. A variety of flavours will get your baby used to different things.

The timings given opposite are just a guide - let your baby set the pace. In general, you want to try to introduce these food groups in the first 2 months of weaning. If you have any food allergies in the family, you might want to wait until the baby is 1 year before you try introducing those foods, or speak with your doctor first.

Once your baby is 6 months (not before) work through the following food groups step by step.

1. Veggies

An Italian nutritionist gave me the best advice for my first weaning dish when she introduced me to Baby Brodino. This is a veggie broth that is super-simple to make (using 3 vegetables) and can be adapted to introduce other flavours easily – you just boil a carrot, a potato and a courgette in water and blitz (see page 68). After a few days of making it this way, you can mix up the vegetables, and later on you can add meats and other ingredients to the same dish (a spoon of olive oil and a scoop of Parmesan). So from day 1, you have a simple Italian solution which can stay with you for the whole Step A of weaning.

My other tip for purées on the go is my Pick 'n' Mix Cubes (see page 74). Make some basic veg or fruit purées (see page 70) and freeze them in ice-cube trays. You can then 'pick 'n' mix' from a selection in your freezer when you're on the run and easily vary meals.

2. Meat, fish and eggs

Keep preparing your Baby Brodino and add the following meats to it, one at a time . . . Introduce white meat (chicken/turkey) and fish first – I started with cod, hake, salmon and tuna, and in later weeks introduced stronger flavours such as mackerel and sardines (in small amounts, as these fish are saltier). Next, introduce red meats (beef, veal, lamb) and eggs.

You can also add steamed/cooked meats or fish to your Pick 'n' Mix Cubes. Just make sure all the ingredients are cooked fully (see page 73 for advice on reheating, etc.).

3. Gluten and nuts

Now introduce gluten into your baby's diet. This is usually kept until last, as there is a higher risk of allergies when introducing gluten – toast or rusks are a great starting point (see page 92).

When it comes to introducing nuts, you should obviously not give whole nuts because of the risk of choking – however, ground nuts are a fantastic source of nutrients and a great addition to any purée. If you have any evidence of allergies to gluten or nuts in your family, you might want to wait until the baby is at least 1 year old before introducing these foods, or speak with your doctor.

The image labels read: **WEEKS 1-4**, **WEEKS 5-6**, **WEEKS 7-8**.

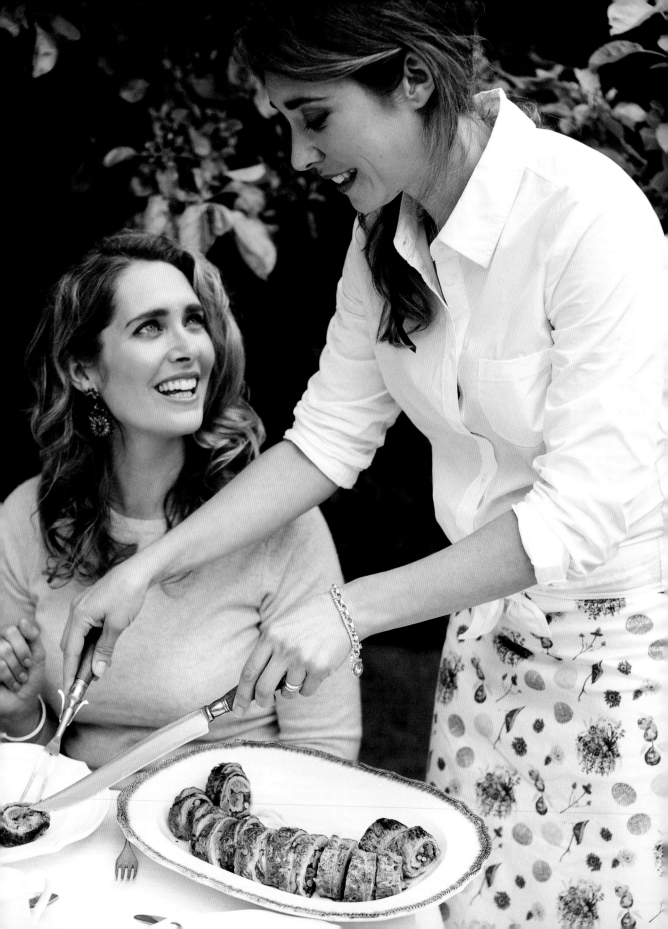

SECRETS OF SUCCESS

Happy mum = happy child.
Easier said than done, I know, but try to relax when it comes to weaning and feeding your kids. There will often be battles, tantrums and rejection of certain foods, but try not to make a fuss about it. Ignore it, and try again another day. Sometimes it can take about 5 or 10 attempts to get a baby used to a new flavour. Remember, babies get all the nutrition they need from milk in the early stages of weaning, so let them explore, be curious and be happy.

Variety is key.
From 6–8 months, weaning is less about nutrition and more about taste, variety and changes in texture. The quicker you can introduce variety the better – try mixing up colours of fruit and veg, different carbs, fats and proteins, herbs and spices. Vary the temperatures too . . . warm and cold. This is the easiest time to explore variety, and the more you mix it up the less likely it is that your child will be a picky eater later on. Try giving the same vegetable in lots of different ways – whole, finely chopped, puréed, etc. (For inspiration, see page 110.) Also, you need to start giving texture quickly, because by 9 months a baby is more likely to reject lumps if she has had only blended purées up until then.

Get ahead essentials.
If you want to make your life easy in the kitchen, see pages 22–33; this will save you precious time when cooking baby and family meals. These 3 simple essentials (Freezer, Equipment and Store cupboard) will transform you into Super-Mum!

Confidence.

Don't be scared, especially when weaning – trust your instinct. Choking is definitely a concern when feeding your children, but provided you take the weaning stage step by step, nature has an amazing way of allowing your child to progress. Never leave your children unattended when eating, but enjoy letting them explore tastes and textures.

Keep it simple.

Lots of weaning guides are hugely detailed, and some talk about specific weeks for introducing vegetables and fruits. And many offer contradictory advice. National guidelines actually say that, as of 6 months, a baby can eat almost anything (see the list of foods to avoid on page 40).

The pleasure of eating.

Help children see food and eating as a fun thing to do – not an obligation. This is why weaning at 6 months is fantastic. There's no major rush . . . the first meals are an introduction to flavours and to the pleasure of eating, rather than being concerned with quantity, as milk is still the baby's main source of nutrition. So relax and have fun. Let your baby set the pace. Just as we don't tell a baby when they should start to crawl or walk, let them set the pace when it comes to food too. We can encourage certain mealtimes and a portion size, but you should let your baby be your guide. They'll tell you if they want more or have had enough.

Pick a good time.

Avoid weaning if your baby is tired or hungry, and pick a time of day when you are relaxed and not too rushed. It is more important that you are both in good spirits – whether at breakfast, lunch or dinner.

If you fail, try again.

Some doctors say it can take up to 10 tries of the same food before it is accepted, so don't give up. Also, if a baby spits food out, wrinkles her nose or scrunches up her face, that doesn't necessarily mean she doesn't like the food . . . Don't give up after the first go, keep trying!

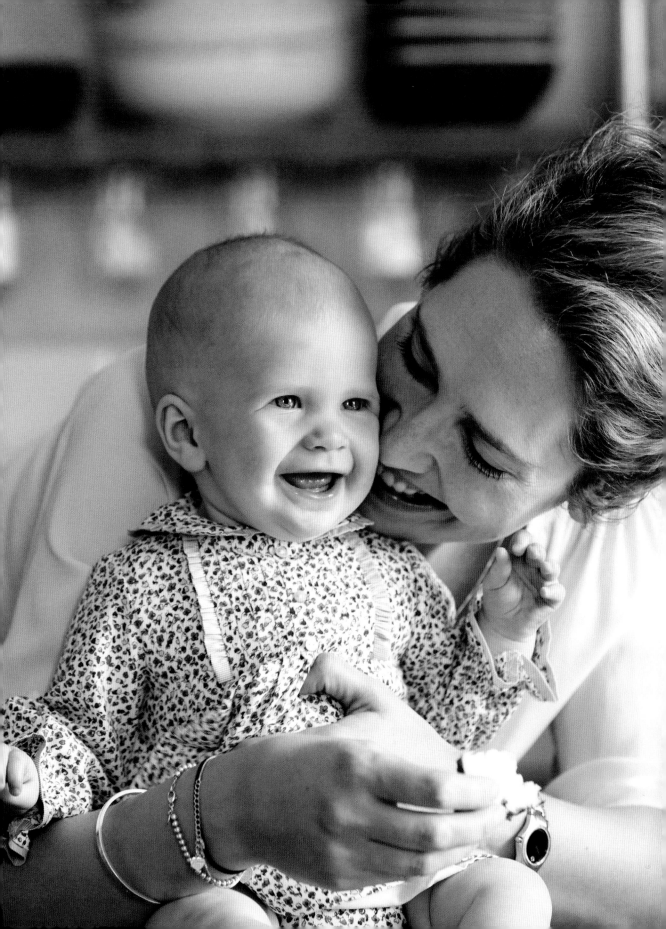

HOW I DID IT

Here are some nuggets and tips
that really worked for me.

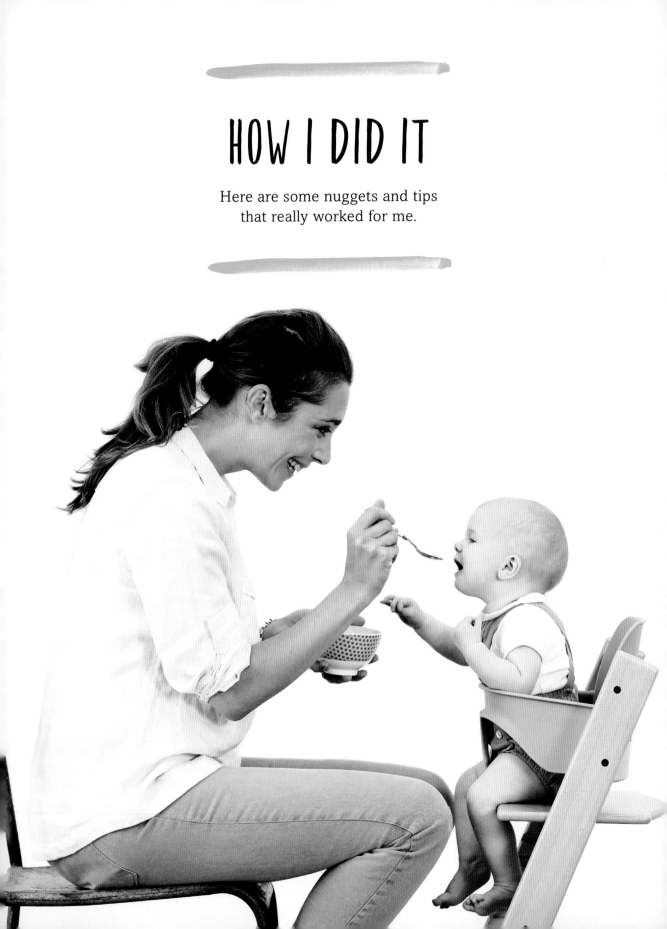

Keeping breakfast the same.
Our nonna always said it's a really good plan to keep breakfast as simple and consistent as possible (see page 49).

Brodino at home.
I found making Baby Brodino was one of the easiest meals when at home (see page 68). It's easy to do, and I'd throw in a range of veggies each day to mix it up. Easy to add some meat or extra protein too.

Finger foods vs. purées.
Before every meal, I always used to give my little one a selection of finger foods. It kept her occupied while I was preparing her purée, and allowed her to explore new flavours and textures (see page 86 for ideas), as well as improving her pincer grip and hand-eye coordination. However, I liked to make sure a purée was always offered so that I could be sure she had eaten something.

Mix 'n' match when out and about.
When going out and about, I found choosing some Pick 'n' Mix Cubes from the freezer the easiest thing to do (see page 74). Grab and go, and easy to heat up if on the run. They can also be eaten at room temperature/cool – I think it's good to get your baby used to different food temperatures (just make sure the purée you give has already been fully cooked prior to freezing).

Snacks not necessary.
Snacks are a brilliant way to distract your baby or calm her down (and I regularly tear open the bread when going around the supermarket to give me some peace), but feeling the need to provide a regular snack between every meal is not necessary, in my opinion. The more we train our kids to get used to a snack, the more they will demand it. Offer snacks at irregular times during the day or avoid them where possible.

No dessert.
I've tried not to fall into the trap of always offering dessert. It seems something we are programmed to do as adults (to have our sweet treat after food), but it really isn't necessary, and I didn't want my kids getting into the habit of not eating their main and always expecting a dessert.

First fruit or veg?
There are lots of opinions out there about whether it's best to wean with fruit or veg first. I don't think it really matters . . . at 6 months a baby can eat most things, so don't spend your days stressing about the detail. Encourage as many veggies as possible and limit the sweet treats. Also, at 6 months, babies are more accepting of bitter flavours from green veg than after 8 months, so take advantage! It has often been argued that giving a baby a sweeter fruit or veg as a first food may lead them to develop a sweet tooth and potentially reject more bitter veggies further down the line. The best advice is to try and avoid starting off with a very sweet fruit.

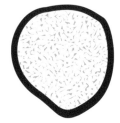
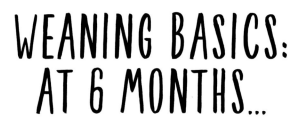

WEANING BASICS:
AT 6 MONTHS...

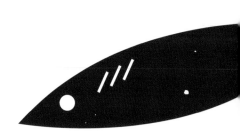

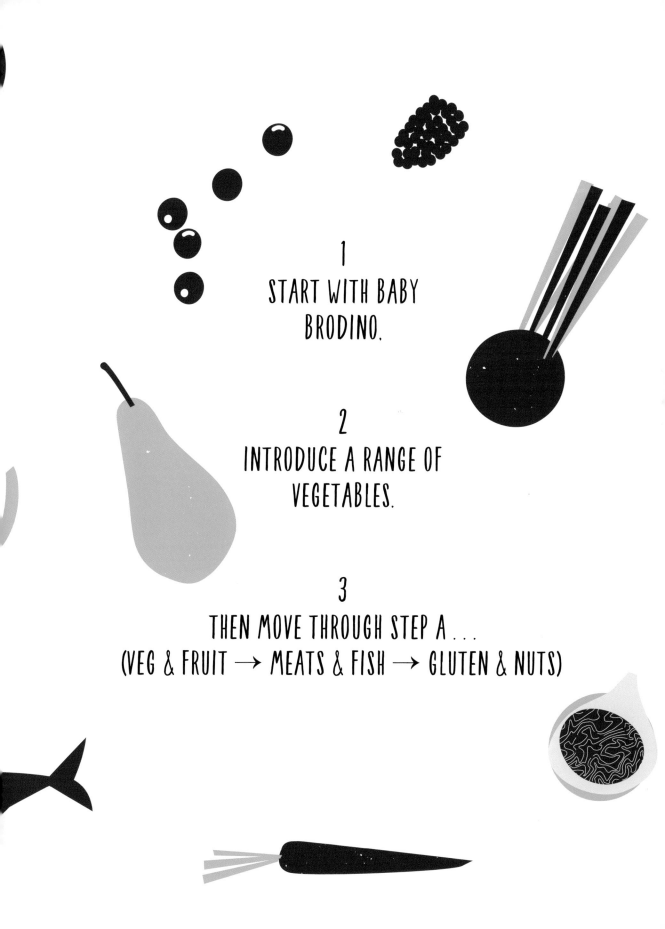

1
START WITH BABY BRODINO.

2
INTRODUCE A RANGE OF VEGETABLES.

3
THEN MOVE THROUGH STEP A . . .
(VEG & FRUIT → MEATS & FISH → GLUTEN & NUTS)

BABY BRODINO

This baby broth (brodino) is the best and easiest way to start weaning your baby. It was recommended to me by an Italian nutritionist, and after months of stressing about how to start, and what to give my baby, this recipe was so simple and invaluable. I would recommend any parent starting to wean their baby to begin with Baby Brodino.

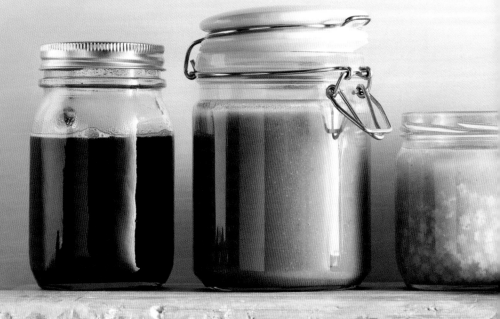

DIFFERENT VEGETABLES

Always keep 1 potato in the recipe, but change the other vegetables.

For example, try swapping the carrot and courgette for parsnip, cauliflower, sweet potato, broccoli, pepper, celery or beetroot.

It's also great to swap one of the vegetables for a fruit (apple, pear, mango, etc.).

FLAVOURS

Introduce different herbs/spices/flavours:

Baby Brodino + 1 teaspoon of olive oil
                          and grated Parmesan
Baby Brodino + a sprinkling of paprika
Baby Brodino + basil

BASE RECIPE

This makes a large quantity that will last for a couple of days (in the fridge) and can also be frozen (see page 25 for how to freeze).

1 small potato
1 carrot
1 courgette

Peel your veg and chop into small cubes.

Cover the veg with water and boil until soft.

Drain off the water but don't throw it away.

Purée the vegetables.

Add some of the reserved water to loosen or thicken to the desired consistency.

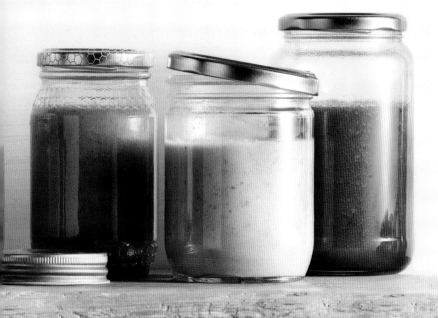

GLUTEN/NUTS

Baby Brodino + pastina
Baby Brodino + ground almonds
Baby Brodino + breadcrumbs

Ultimately you can vary all the flavours, textures and tastes using this method, to get your baby used to a whole range of foods.

MEAT/FISH

Introduce meat and fish.

Boil the meat/fish at the same time as your veg and blend together:

Baby Brodino + portion of chicken
Baby Brodino + portion of minced beef
Baby Brodino + portion of cod/salmon

MAKING A BASIC PURÉE

How to steam, how to purée and how to thicken

HOW TO STEAM YOUR BABY'S FOOD

The most effective way of cooking your baby's food is to steam it. Steaming food means it keeps in the maximum nutrients and flavours. Steaming fruit and veg so they are just soft, rather than mushy, is best – it retains more flavour and encourages the baby to get used to texture. When steaming meat or fish, make sure it is fully cooked.

There are different methods of steaming your food:

1. Quick and minimal washing up
Microwave – the quickest way to steam your veg. Put your ingredients into a bowl and pour over a little water. Cover with clingfilm, pierce the film with a few holes, then microwave until soft according to the microwave manufacturer's instructions.

2. Old-school way
Saucepan + steamer basket (or stainless-steel colander). Put some water in your saucepan, then place your steamer basket or colander on top. Put your ingredients inside the basket/colander, cover with a lid, and turn on the heat until cooked through. Make sure the lid forms a closed seal over the colander and keeps the steam in. Keep checking the water hasn't dried up or you'll end up with a burnt pan.

3. Fancy but bulky
Steamer tower – there are different versions available to buy, so do read the various reviews. The downside is that they can be more expensive and take up quite a bit of space in your kitchen – and need more washing up.

HOW TO PURÉE

For me, the ultimate kitchen gadget you MUST have when weaning your baby (or indeed feeding a family) is a stick blender. There's no need for an expensive food processor. Stick blenders are economical but also small and neat, so are easy to store. I would recommend buying one with a pot attachment. Quite simply you use the blender to blitz your purée to the desired consistency, adding milk or water to loosen.

This is the easiest way to blend your purées (and it's super-versatile for making pestos, soups, smoothies, ice lollies and other great recipes for later years too).

Other options include: a masher or ricer (difficult to get a smooth consistency), or a food processor (large, bulky and expensive, plus lots of washing up).

HOW THICK?

A first purée should be similar to non-set yoghurt: it should be thick enough to be picked up easily on a spoon, but thin enough to drop off the spoon (like honey).

If your purée is too thick, loosen it with your baby's usual milk or cooled boiled water.

If your purée is too runny, add more food or a spoonful of baby rice.

Try to vary the texture of your purées as early as possible to prevent your baby becoming a picky eater later on.

HOW TO FREEZE A BASIC PURÉE

HOW TO FREEZE AND STORE

Once your purée is fully cooled, pour it into ice-cube trays.

Place in the freezer until solid.

Once solid, remove the ice cubes - to help you do this, run hot water over the base of your ice-cube tray, or place it on a baking tray and pour boiling water round the ice-cube tray to release the cubes.

Place the frozen cubes in freezer bags to free up your ice-cube tray and also minimize on storage space (always label your freezer bag so you know what purée the bag contains, and make sure it has a date on it too).

HOW TO DEFROST/REHEAT

Defrosting
The safest ways to defrost are in the fridge overnight and using a microwave.

Make sure your food is completely defrosted before you reheat it.

Never refreeze food that has already been frozen and defrosted.

Reheating
Cook food so it's piping hot, then cool to a lukewarm temperature - you can use a microwave or pan.

Don't ever reheat food more than once.

Always make sure the food is completely cooled before putting it into the fridge or freezer.

HOW HOT?

Always stir your purée before testing the heat (especially if heated in a microwave), to get rid of 'hot spots'.

Always test the food on the inside of your wrist - it should feel neither hot nor cold.

PICK 'N' MIX CUBES

Pick 'n' Mix Cubes are a brilliantly easy way to vary your baby's meals on the go. I prepare a range of different flavoured purées at the weekend, freeze them in cubes, bag them up in my freezer, and then, when I am going out and about, pick and mix flavours by the day.

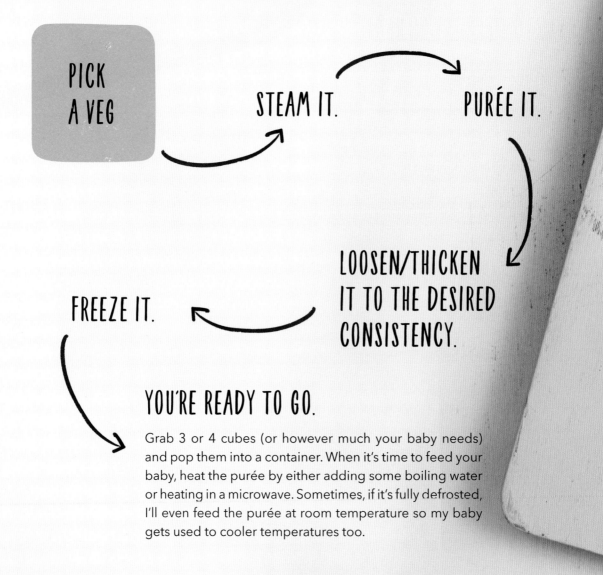

PICK A VEG → **STEAM IT.** → **PURÉE IT.**

LOOSEN/THICKEN IT TO THE DESIRED CONSISTENCY.

FREEZE IT.

YOU'RE READY TO GO.

Grab 3 or 4 cubes (or however much your baby needs) and pop them into a container. When it's time to feed your baby, heat the purée by either adding some boiling water or heating in a microwave. Sometimes, if it's fully defrosted, I'll even feed the purée at room temperature so my baby gets used to cooler temperatures too.

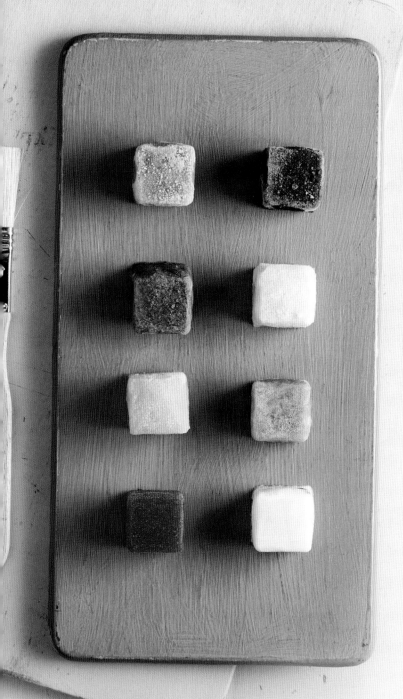

In my freezer I usually stock a range of the following:

Veg purées
e.g. pea, parsnip, sweet potato, pepper, broccoli, potato.

Meat and fish purées
e.g. a fish such as cod or salmon, a white meat such as chicken or turkey, a red meat such as beef or lamb.

Fruit purées
e.g. apple, pear, plum, pineapple, mango.

Tips: Don't stress about having a purée for every veg/ingredient under the sun. I usually try to have about 4 veg, 1 meat, 1 fish and 2 fruit purées in the freezer.

Always take your purées out of the ice-cube tray and pop them into a freezer bag once frozen, to reduce the amount of space they take up (and to free up your ice-cube tray!).

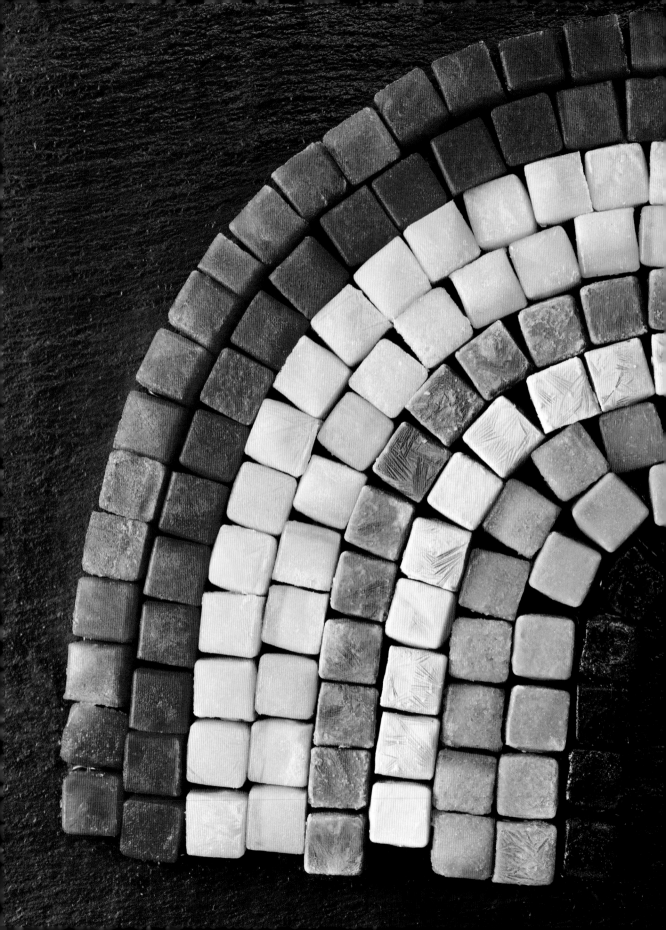

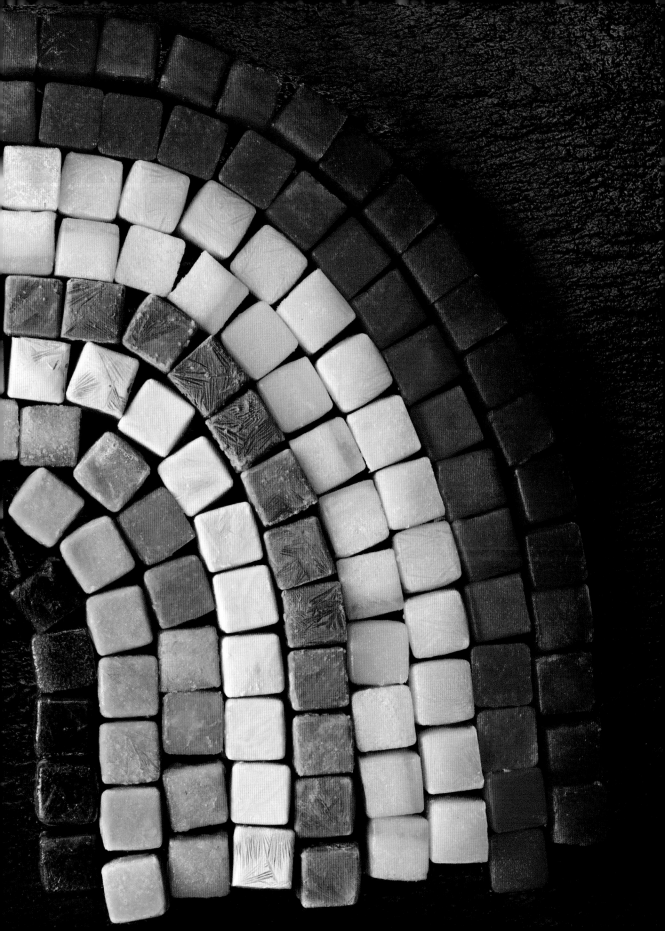

FRUIT AND VEG

Here are some flavour ideas for your first fruit and veg purées.
You can mix things up as you like but these are some of our
favourite combinations. We tend to use equal quantities of veg
and fruit and then vary the liquid and herbs to personal
preference. For how to cook a basic purée, see page 70.

Carrot, potato and milk

1 small carrot, peeled
½ small potato, peeled
a splash of milk

Courgette, carrot and mint

½ small courgette
1 small carrot, peeled
1 sprig of mint

Broccoli, sweet potato and basil

2 broccoli florets
½ small sweet potato, peeled
2 basil leaves

Cauliflower, apple and sweet potato

2 cauliflower florets
½ apple, peeled
½ small sweet potato, peeled

Spinach, date and yoghurt

a handful of spinach
1 date, pitted
1 tbsp plain yoghurt

Pear and yoghurt

1 ripe pear
2 tbsp plain yoghurt

Carrot, apple and oats

1 small carrot, peeled
½ apple
1 tbsp oats

Ricotta, apple and cinnamon

2 tbsp ricotta
½ apple
½ tsp cinnamon

Raspberry, pear and apple

a handful of raspberries
½ pear
½ apple

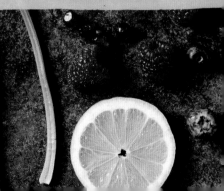

Sweet combinations are great for adults too – serve warm over ice cream or yoghurt.

Most savoury purées are great for adults – leave chunky, add seasoning and serve with olive oil and chilli flakes over pasta or as a dip.

MEAT AND FISH

Here are some flavour ideas for your first meat and fish purées. You can mix things up as you like but these are some of our favourite combinations. We tend to use equal quantities of veg, fruit, meat and fish and then vary the liquid and herbs to personal preference. For cooking purées, see page 70.

Beef, apple and sage

50–80g beef, minced
½ apple
1 sage leaf

Beef, sweet potato and ricotta

50–80g beef, minced
½ sweet potato, peeled
1 tbsp ricotta

Chicken, potato and apple

50–80g chicken
½ small potato, peeled
½ apple

Chicken, butternut squash and ginger

50–80g chicken
50–80g butternut squash, peeled
¼ tsp ground ginger

Turkey and parsnip

50–80g turkey
1 small parsnip

Cod, sweet potato and paprika

50–80g cod
½ small sweet potato, peeled
¼ tsp paprika

Salmon, broccoli and lemon

50–80g salmon
2 broccoli florets
a squirt of lemon juice

Hake, sweet potato and peas

50–80g hake
½ sweet potato, peeled
a handful of peas

Chicken, avocado and basil

50–80g chicken
½ avocado
2 basil leaves

GLUTEN AND NUTS

Here are some flavour ideas for your first gluten and nut purées. You can mix things up as you like but these are some of our favourite combinations. We tend to use equal quantities of the main ingredients (veg/fruit/nuts/pasta) and then vary the liquid and herbs to personal preference. For cooking purées, see page 70.

Pastina, peas, spinach and mint

a handful of pastina
a handful of peas
a handful of spinach
a sprig of mint

Pasta, ham and cheese

a handful of pasta
2 slices of ham
a handful of cheese

Apple, ricotta and walnuts

½ apple
1 tbsp ricotta
2-3 walnuts

Mango, cashews and yoghurt

½ mango
a small handful of cashews
1 tbsp yoghurt

Kiwi, pistachio and avocado

1 kiwi
½ avocado
a small handful of pistachios

Oats, banana and blueberry

a handful of oats
½ banana
a handful of blueberries

Avocado, cucumber and pine nuts

½ avocado
1 piece of cucumber
a handful of pine nuts

Peach, coconut milk and ground almonds

1 ripe peach
a splash of coconut milk
a handful of ground almonds

Blueberry, pear, ground almonds and yoghurt

a handful of blueberries
½ pear
a handful of ground almonds
1 tbsp yoghurt

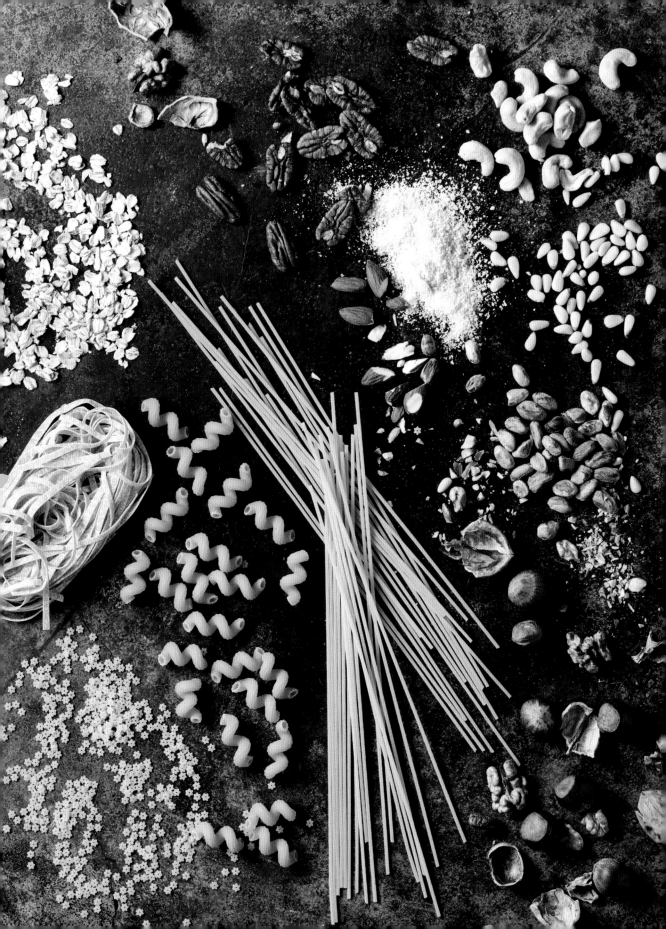

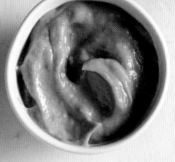

MANGO, GINGER AND YOGHURT

BEETROOT, GROUND ALMONDS AND RICOTTA

NO-COOK PURÉES

These are a brilliantly easy way to prepare food at lightening speed...just throw a handful of each ingredient into a blender and job done!

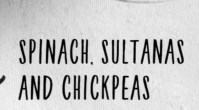

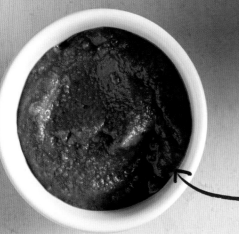

SPINACH, SULTANAS AND CHICKPEAS

You can loosen your no-cook purees with a splash of milk, olive oil or water to reach the desired consistency.

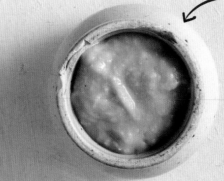

BEANS, SWEETCORN AND SPINACH

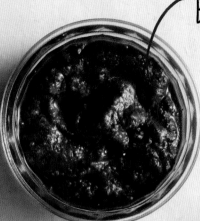

BLUEBERRY AND CHICKPEA

BUTTERBEAN
AND SPINACH

Great for adults: add
seasoning and serve
as a dip.

RED PEPPER AND
CANNELLINI BEANS

TUNA AND CANNELLINI BEANS

BANANA
AND KALE

AVOCADO, FIG
AND SPINACH

Great for adults: add
seasoning and serve
as a dip.

HARD-BOILED
EGGS

POMEGRANATE
SEEDS

KIWI

PEAS

GRATED
MOZZARELLA

FINGER FOODS

SWEETCORN

BLUEBERRIES

PEPPERS

COOKED SWEET
POTATOES

COOKED
SPAGHETTI

TEETHING IDEAS

FROZEN MANGO STONE

BANANA TEETHING RUSKS (SEE PAGE 92)

FROZEN MUSLIN SOAKED IN CAMOMILE

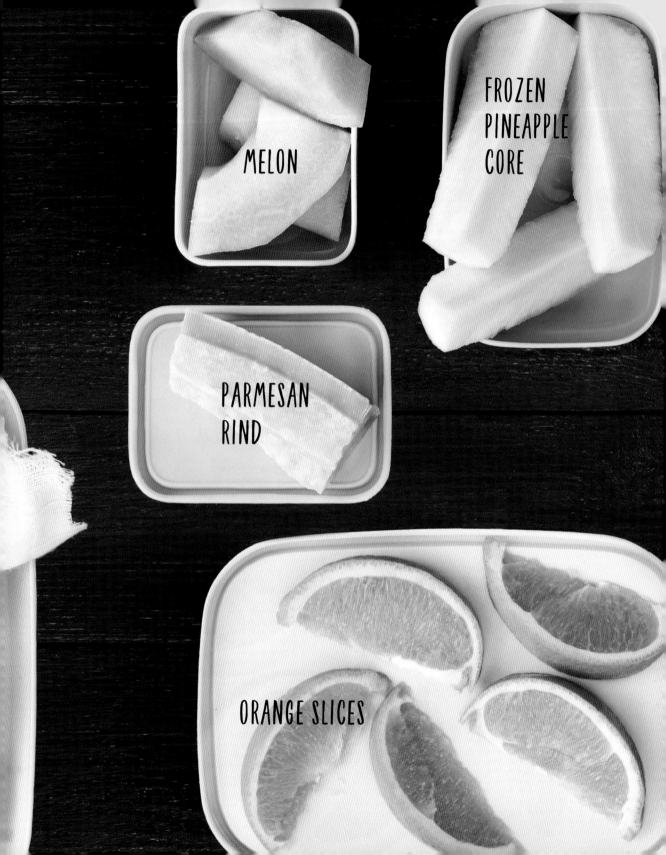

MELON

FROZEN
PINEAPPLE
CORE

PARMESAN
RIND

ORANGE SLICES

MASKING IT TIPS

Here are some great ways to hide extra goodies in your recipes:

CHEAT'S WHITE SAUCE:

ricotta, loosened with milk to desired thickness, seasoned with salt (omit if cooking for a baby), pepper and nutmeg

SUPER BEAN CREAM:

blitz a tin of cannellini beans to a paste and loosen with a splash of milk

KALE CRUMBS:

raw blitzed kale (see page 26)

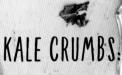

SECRET SPRINKLES:
(SEE PAGE 157)

FOOL'S MAYO:

2 tablespoons Greek
yoghurt, a squirt of
lemon juice and a
teaspoon of olive oil

BEETROOT BLITZ:

roasted beetroot, blitzed

BANANA TEETHING RUSKS

Preparation time: 10 minutes
Cooking time: 15–20 minutes
Makes: 18–20

Store-cupboard essentials:
100g plain flour
2 tablespoons olive oil
4–6 tablespoons water

To buy:
1 ripe banana
100g baby rice cereal

Preheat the oven to 200°C/gas 6.

Line a baking tray with a silicone mat or parchment paper.

Mash the peeled banana in a bowl.

Mix in the rice cereal, flour and oil.

Add a tablespoon of the water at a time until a soft dough is formed.

Roll into finger-size batons, place on a baking tray and press with your finger to flatten them slightly.

Bake for 15–20 minutes, until golden brown.

Leave to cool completely.

Store in an airtight container in the fridge for 2–3 days.

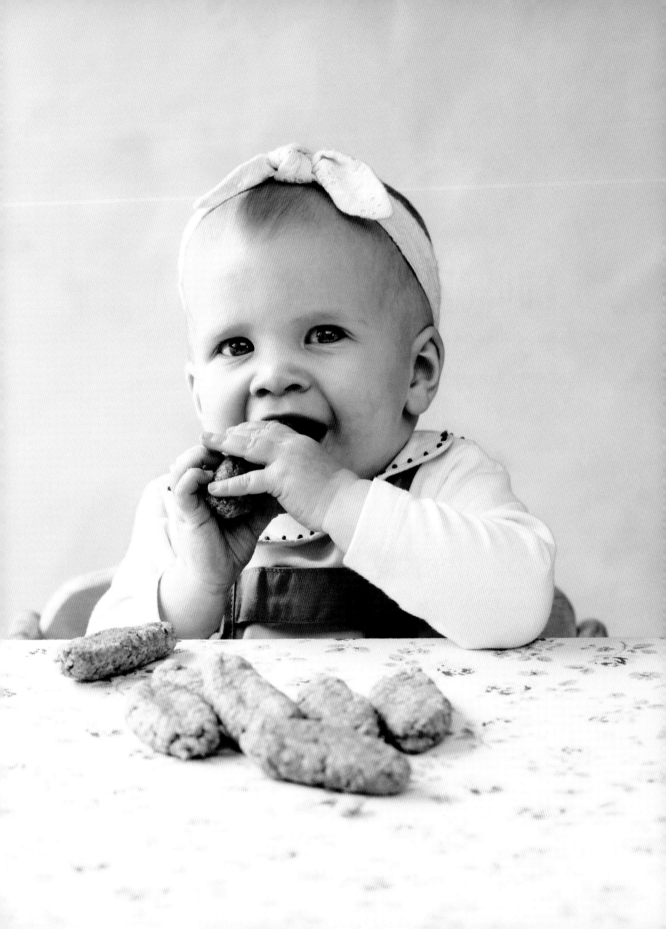

COURGETTE FAMILY PASTA

Preparation time: 5 minutes
Cooking time: according to pasta packet instructions
Serves: 1–2 babies

Bring the water to the boil in a saucepan over a medium heat and add your pastina.

Grate your courgette.

Lower the heat once the pasta is half cooked and add the grated courgette.

Add the egg yolk, Parmesan and olive oil after a couple of minutes.

Reduce the broth to a simmer so that it thickens and most of the water is absorbed.

Cool before serving.

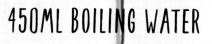
450ML BOILING WATER

1 TABLESPOON GRATED
PARMESAN

2 HANDFULS
OF PASTINA

1 EGG YOLK

1 TABLESPOON
OLIVE OIL

1 COURGETTE

PASTA, CARROT AND RICOTTA

Preparation time: 5 minutes
Cooking time: according to pasta packet instructions
Serves: 1–2 babies

Bring the water to the boil in a saucepan over a medium heat and add the pastina.

Grate the carrot. When the pasta has almost absorbed all the water, add your grated carrot and cook for a few more minutes, until the carrot has softened.

Remove from the heat and place in a bowl.

Add the ricotta, and mix together until well combined.

Season with the Parmesan to taste.

1 SMALL CARROT,
PEELED

A HANDFUL
OF PASTINA
(SMALL PASTA)

225ML
WATER

1 TABLESPOON
OF RICOTTA

GRATED
PARMESAN

BEEF, PARSNIP, APPLE AND CINNAMON

Preparation time: 5 minutes
Cooking time: 15 minutes
Serves: 1–2 babies

Store-cupboard essentials:
a drizzle of extra virgin olive oil

Cut the parsnip and apple into small pieces.

Steam the beef, parsnip and apple in a steamer for 10-15 minutes, until the beef is cooked through and the parsnip and apple are soft throughout.

Add the cinnamon and olive oil, then either blitz with a stick blender for a small baby or mash with a fork for an older baby.

50-80G MINCED BEEF

1 SMALL APPLE

1 SMALL PARSNIP

½ TEASPOON GROUND
CINNAMON

BEETROOT, PEACH AND COCONUT

Preparation time: 2 minutes
Serves: 1–2 babies

Blend all the ingredients together until completely smooth and no lumps are left.

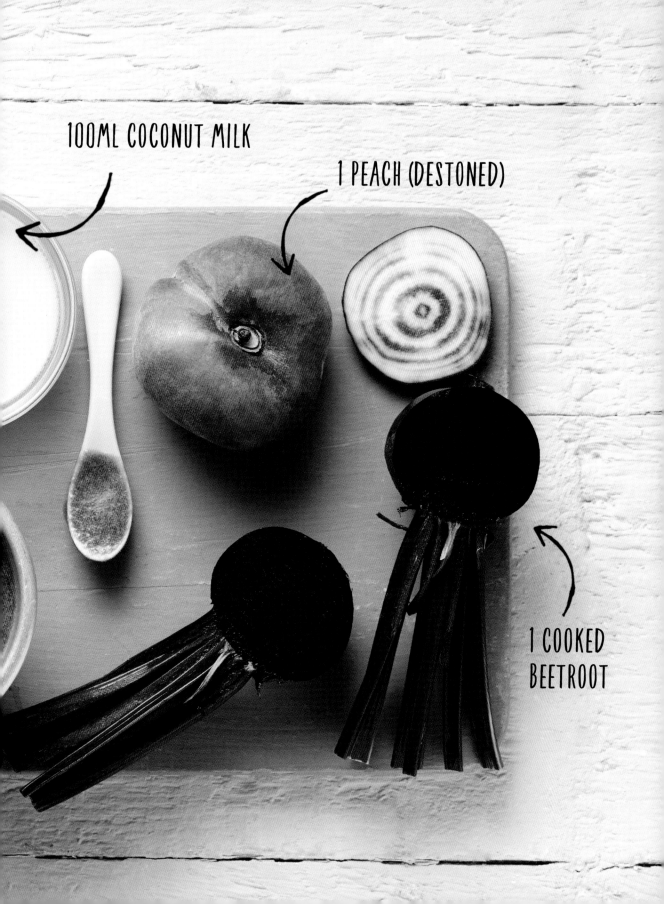

100ML COCONUT MILK

1 PEACH (DESTONED)

1 COOKED
BEETROOT

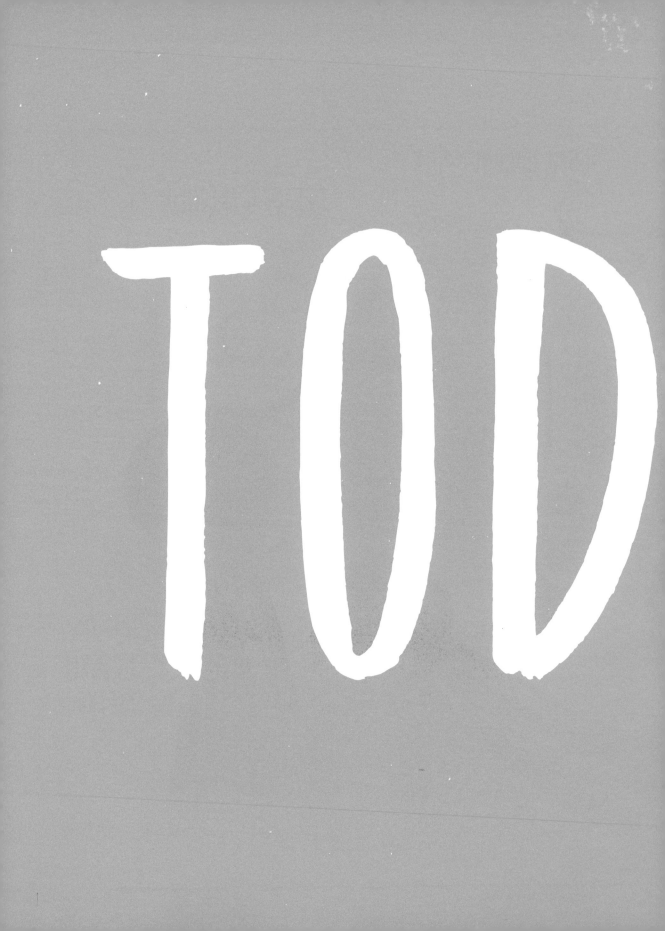

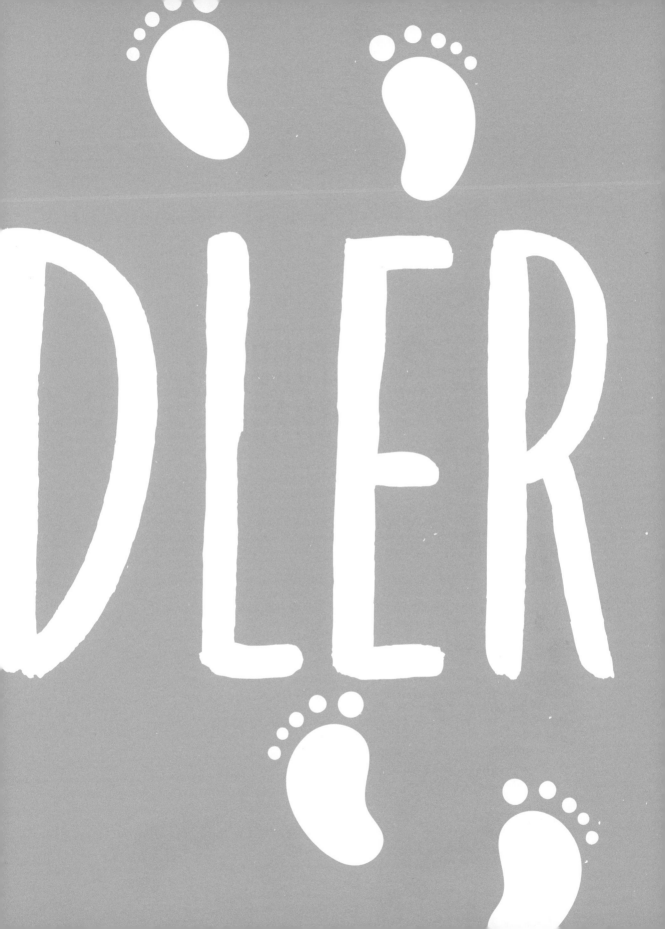

TODDLER: SNACKS

The most important and yet most difficult time when it comes to feeding your children and preventing them becoming picky eaters, is the terrible 2s. So many parents have told me that their children ate everything as babies, but by 2 or 3 years old it changed and now all they touch is square pieces of toast, ham sandwiches or potatoes.

Sound familiar?

I witnessed this with my little girl; 2 was the age when she started to assert herself. She knew what she liked and what she didn't like and boy, oh boy, did she tell me. Suddenly, after months of glugging Greek yoghurt, she no longer wanted to touch the stuff and would become very cautious about anything white in colour.

The most important time to prevent picky eaters and yet the biggest hurdle . . . 2-year-olds.

But this is the time to stand your ground . . . it's the most important time to tell them who's boss. If you give in now, you're likely to start going down one long slippery slope. So on the next few pages I've listed some tips to help you gain some inner will-power.

I've also been told by other mums that the toddler stage is the most challenging when it comes to mealtimes. Kids get tired and usually hungry at the same time, so while eating one meal with the family is the ideal, often a clingy, hungry child wins the battle on the snack/separate meal front. So this chapter is also about giving you quick-fix yet healthy snack ideas (to keep them going until dinnertime) and speedy emergency recipes for getting quick lunch meals on the table to avoid the tantrums.

Ultimately this chapter is all about the speedy lunchtime meal, travel or lunchbox solution and quick-fix snacks. Basically anything that can act as a filler until your family mealtime.

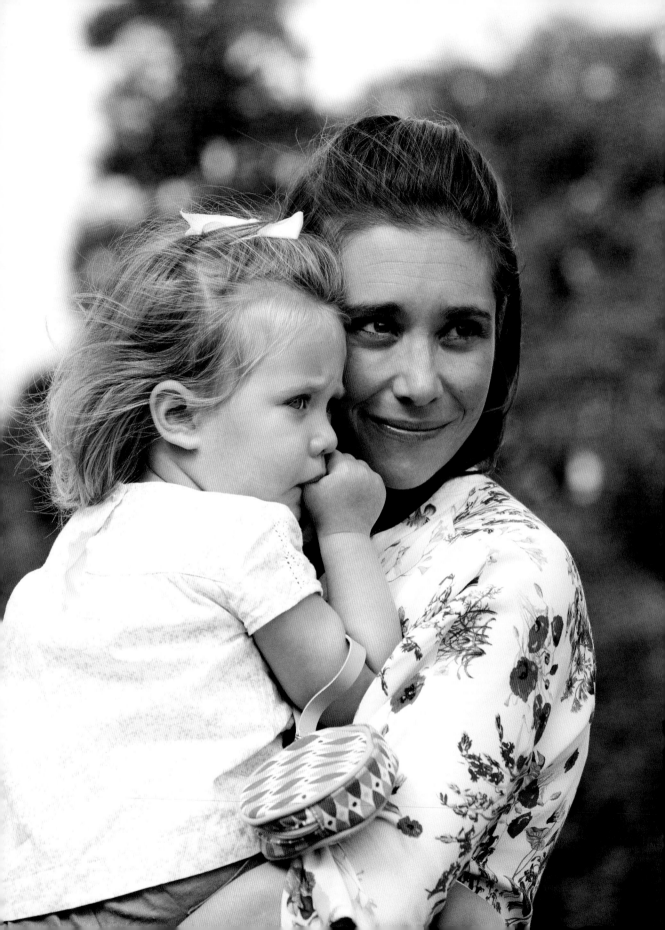

SECRETS OF SUCCESS

One option only.

Toddlers are clever cookies, and the minute you start giving in to them, you've had your chips! Provided they are in full health, the best advice I could give you is do not offer substitutes. Decide before you dish up what you're going to offer as a meal and don't back down. If it doesn't get eaten, don't make a fuss, just move on. If nothing gets eaten, then so be it. Kids are super clever, and the minute they see you giving in, or grabbing that piece of toast as a substitute, they'll think they've hit the jackpot. The facts you need to consider are that most toddlers overeat – they only need to eat meals the size of their small fist, so they usually have plenty in them to survive missing the odd meal. Think of what happens when they get a little ill . . . they'll often not eat for several days. So, while it goes completely against any mum's natural instinct, try to find the power to be strong and avoid giving in to any signs of a picky eater – I hate any evening I put my little girl to bed without dinner, but it was my husband who helped me stay strong, reassuring me that her oversized belly would keep her fuelled overnight. Toddlers do not need that substitute piece of toast.

Keep up the variety.

Don't obsess about this, but try to make sure you're still offering your kids lots of different flavours and textures throughout the week. We all, including me, fall into the trap of cooking the things we are used to, or meals that are quick (pasta, bread, finger foods, etc.), but every 2–3 days, think what new foods you can give. Or choose a favourite food and cook it a different way (e.g. instead of raw carrot, try roasting it).

Finger foods. Blitzed soups. Combi meals.

Try to offer meals based on these three styles – finger foods, blitzed soups and combi meals (recipes like casseroles or curries, which have rice or other carb mixed up with chunky veg or meat and a sauce). I realized one week that I had been really busy and had been giving my daughter lots of finger foods for several days (basically quick and easy to grab from the fridge), and when I offered her a chunky soup she flat out refused it (despite loving it only a few weeks ago!). I realized that my busy life had led me to neglect giving her different styles of meals and she had started to become picky! Aaaaargh, panic! So I reverted to this 3-meal principle. I gave her the same soup she had rejected 3 meals in a row … After the third attempt, she wolfed it down. And from then on I always tried to mix up the style of meal. Lunches are often finger foods, as they're easier, but then I do chunky soups on some days, smooth soups on others and lots of combi meals. I'm pleased to say that this picky hurdle has been overcome!

Sweet surprise.

I make sure I don't give a dessert after every meal. I found that if I did this too regularly, the kids became accustomed to it and would sometimes reject their meal knowing a sweet treat was to follow. So some days I give fruit or yoghurt and other days I don't. Sometimes I give the dessert as an afternoon snack/treat, other times I'll offer cheese after a meal. The less regularity and the more you mix things up the better, so they don't fall into the trap of expecting it every time. I call it my sweet surprise!

Be realistic.

Be realistic: emergencies and delays do happen (especially when kids are involved!) – traffic jams, queues at the shops, pavement tantrums – so don't try to be Super-Mum in these moments. Be realistic and prepare a meal that can be thrown together quickly, or grab something from your freezer supplies. Save that delicious lasagna you had planned for another time. Remember, keep mealtimes as relaxed as possible and don't try to do too much at once.

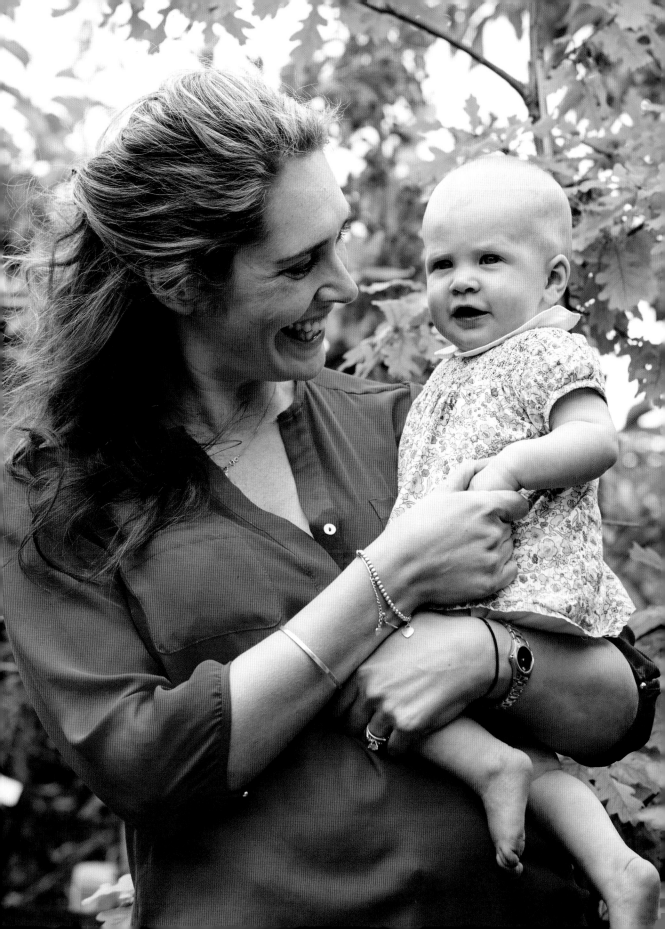

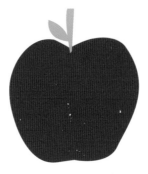

PICK ONE VEG OR FRUIT AND TRY COOKING IT IN MANY DIFFERENT WAYS.

Hot, cold, baked, toasted – don't always
stick to the same thing.

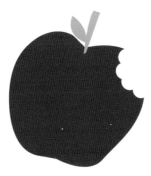

VARIETY. VARIETY. VARIETY.

Pick your kid's favourite veg/fruit
(e.g. an apple) and then mix it up.

BAKE IT

with cinnamon

GRILL IT

with melted cheese

FRY IT

with olive oil and
Cheddar cheese

SPRINKLE IT

grated into porridge
with toasted nuts
and berries

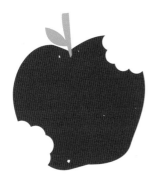

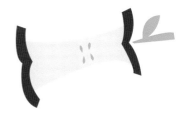

HOW I DID IT

Here are some tips that really worked for me when I started seeing signs of a picky toddler developing.

Mix up foods they love.

Normally my daughter will wolf down porridge, and she absolutely loves raisins as an afternoon snack. (If you are giving dried fruit as a snack remember to serve with water so that it doesn't get stuck in their teeth!) However, when she saw me putting some raisins into her porridge she had a wobbly and picked them all out. Hmm, picky eater alert (and one panicked mum!). Since then I have been mixing some of her favourite foods into the porridge (cinnamon, banana, fruit, raisins). I started by showing her the plain porridge and a pile of raisins separately. Then I asked her to put the raisins into the porridge and stir. She ate it the second time around. My advice – mix and match regular comfort foods as often as possible!

Snacktime flavours.

I love offering my kids new, unusual flavours and seeing what they enjoy or reject. I find the best time to do this is either late morning or just after an afternoon nap (or a time you know they won't be hungry but might be curious and in a good mood).

I don't make a big deal of this and usually I just put the food out in a bowl where they are playing. Sometimes they ignore it, and when they get curious they'll have a taste or lick. Different things I have offered are: flavoured popcorn, warm melted cheese and apple tossed in cinnamon, toasted coconut flakes, chopped pecans and baked sweet potato.

Hidden foods.

If there are foods you are really keen to give your kids (for boosting valuable nutrients), try to find ways to hide them in certain recipes. I am a big believer in educating children to understand what they are eating – however, sometimes you just need a quick fix. There are lots of great ways to do this – try my ideas for Kale Crumbs on page 26 or pink pancakes on page 176.

Same food – different ways.

Make something hot that your child normally eats cold (e.g. an apple). Or to something savoury, add a spice or some sweetness (try grilling some cheese with cinnamon on top). My little one loves raw carrots, so some days I grate them and dress them with olive oil and lemon, other days I'll roast them with garlic. She also loves peaches, so I baked some in the oven with a little butter and maple syrup; she was cautious at first, but then gobbled them up. It's good to get kids used to trying new things as early as possible and learning that new flavours can be tasty too.

Keep persisting without a fuss.

There are some foods my little one has consistently rejected since the weaning days. While she will eat unusual flavours like raw mushrooms, peppers, olives, apricots, mackerel and fennel, she has consistently rejected cherry tomatoes, blueberries, avocado and mango. I will reintroduce them every now and again, but I won't make a fuss if she rejects them. Everyone is entitled to have likes and dislikes. The most important thing is not to make a scene or get angry about it.

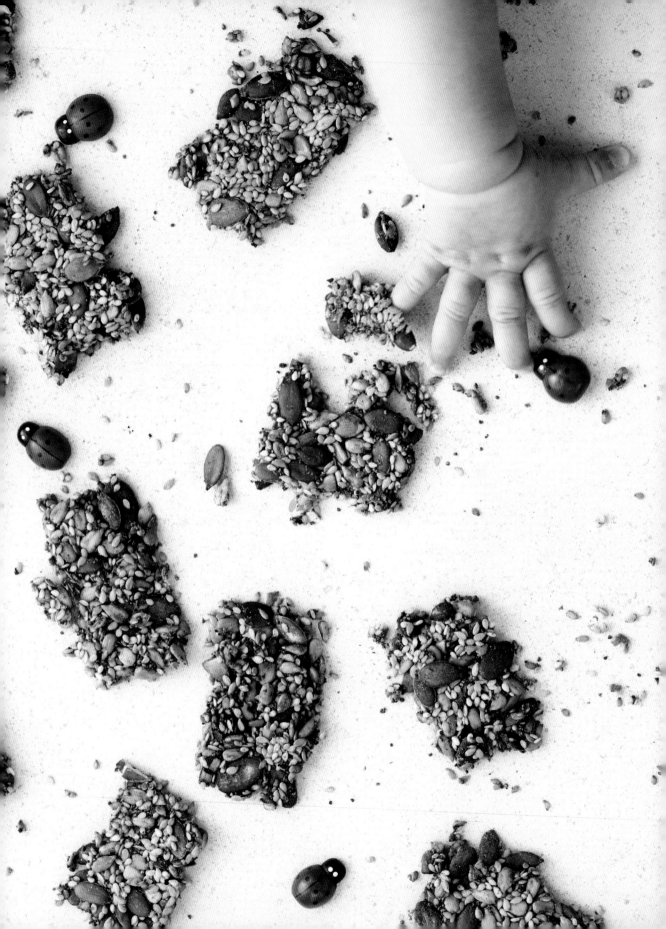

SAVOURY SEED CRACKERS

Preparation time: 10 minutes
Cooking time: 40 minutes
Makes: 12–24 (depending on their size)

To buy:
1 ripe pear (approx. 250g),
   peeled and cored
60g pumpkin seeds
60g sunflower seeds
60g sesame seeds

40g flax seeds
40g chia seeds
15g poppy seeds
1 teaspoon ground nutmeg

Store-cupboard essentials:
1 teaspoon ground cinnamon

Preheat the oven to 180°C/gas 4.

Line a baking tray with parchment paper.

Place the pear in a blender and blitz until puréed.

Mix all the ingredients together in a bowl until everything is well combined.

Scoop the seed mixture on to the parchment paper and spread into a flat, even layer.

Bake for 20 minutes.

Remove from the oven and cut the crackers into rectangles.

Bake for an additional 10-20 minutes, until all the crackers are browned and crispy.

Leave to cool on a wire rack.

Tip: These are best eaten on the day they are made; however, if you don't eat them all and they become a little soft, you can crisp them up again in the oven.

If you're not serving to a baby, you could add a pinch of salt to the mixture.

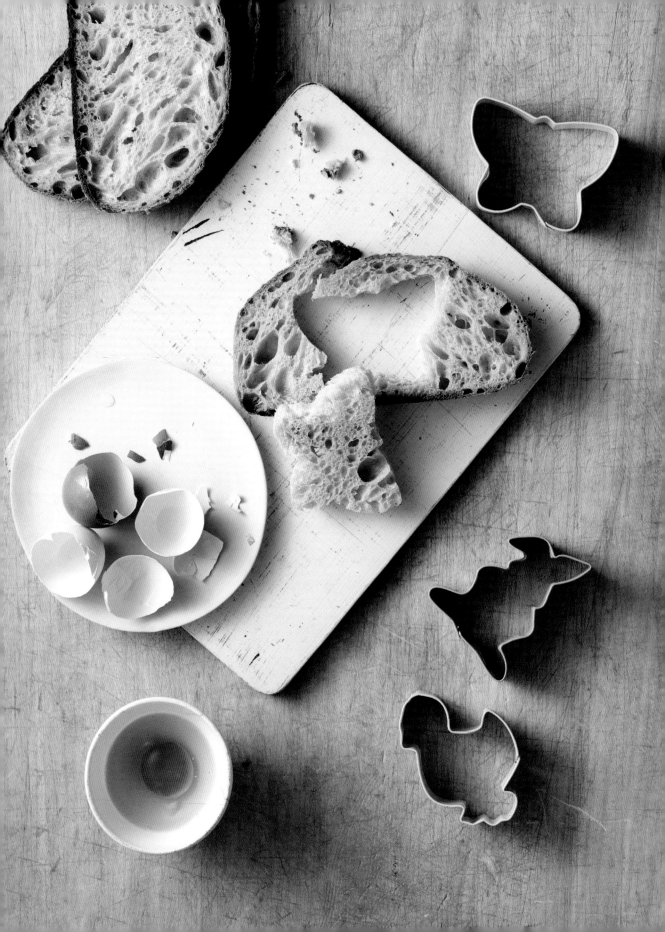

OUR WAY WITH TOAST

Preparation time: 2 minutes
Cooking time: 4–6 minutes
Serves: 4

To buy:
4 slices of bread

Store-cupboard essentials:
butter
4 eggs
salt and pepper, to taste

Cut out the middle of the bread using a shape cutter like a star or a heart.

Heat a frying pan, then add a teaspoon of butter and let it melt.

Place a slice of bread in the pan, then crack an egg into the cut-out middle. Make sure the pan is hot so that the egg doesn't run underneath the bread.

Cook for 2-3 minutes, until most of the egg is cooked through.

Flip the bread and cook on the other side for a further minute until the egg is cooked to your liking.

Season with salt and pepper (for toddlers and adults).

BEETROOT HUMMUS

Preparation time: 5 minutes
Serves: 4

To buy
1 large roasted beetroot
juice of 1 lemon
1 tablespoon tahini

Store-cupboard essentials:
1 x 400g tin of chickpeas
1 clove of garlic
salt, to taste
4 tablespoons extra virgin olive
oil, plus extra to loosen

Drain the chickpeas and rinse.

Blitz all the ingredients until smooth.

Add a splash of olive oil gradually until the hummus has a smooth and creamy texture.

Remove a portion for baby, then season with salt and pepper to taste (for toddlers and adults).

Tips: If you don't have time to roast your beetroot for the Beetroot Blitz, you can blitz it raw.

As an activity to do with kids, let them help remove the skins of the chickpeas - it's not necessary but will make for a smoother hummus.

You can also use kidney, cannellini, butter or borlotti beans if you don't have chickpeas.

SMOKED MACKEREL PÂTÉ

Preparation time: 10 minutes
Serves: 4–6

To buy:
2 smoked mackerel fillets
100g cream cheese
100g crème fraîche
½ a lemon
a handful of chives

Store-cupboard essentials:
pepper, to taste

Skin the mackerel fillets and do a quick check for any bones.

Blend the mackerel, cream cheese and crème fraîche with a stick blender until smooth.

Zest the lemon and squeeze the juice.

Chop the chives.

Mix the chives, lemon zest and juice and pepper into the mackerel mixture.

Tip: Feel free to experiment with other smoked fish like salmon or trout. No extra salt is needed, as smoked fish in general is salty. It is possible to buy lightly smoked fish, which is lower in salt, so keep a lookout for these.

3 HEALTHY WAYS WITH CROQUETTES

Preparation time: 10 minutes
Cooking time: 20–30 minutes

Basic croquette method

Preheat the oven to 200°C/gas 6.

Grease a mini muffin tin (35 x 25cm) with oil and set aside.

Place the veg inside a clean kitchen towel and squeeze out any excess moisture.

Combine all the ingredients in a large bowl and mix together thoroughly.

Scoop a tablespoon of the mixture into each muffin cup and press down firmly.

Bake for 20-30 minutes, or until the croquettes are golden brown.

Baked cauli croquettes

To buy:
½ a cauliflower, blitzed
2 handfuls of grated cheese (we like to use Cheddar) (approx. 80g)
a small handful of polenta/semolina flour (approx. 20g)
½ teaspoon ground mustard

Store-cupboard essentials:
2 eggs
a few grinds of pepper
1 sprig of fresh or dried rosemary
olive oil

Baked courgette croquettes

To buy:
2 courgettes, grated
2 handfuls of grated cheese (we like to use Cheddar) (approx. 80g)
a small handful of polenta/semolina flour (approx. 20g)

Store-cupboard essentials:
2 eggs
a few grinds of pepper
½ teaspoon dried or fresh rosemary
olive oil

Baked sweet potato croquettes

To buy:
1 sweet potato, grated
2 handfuls of crumbled feta cheese (approx. 80g)
a small handful of polenta/semolina flour
½ teaspoon chopped dried or fresh thyme

Store-cupboard essentials:
2 eggs
a few grinds of pepper
olive oil

Each of the above variations follows the same basic method - simply swap the ingredients as necessary.

KALE AND LEMON CREAM CHEESE SPREAD/DIP

Preparation time: 2 minutes
Serves: 6

To buy
200g cream cheese
zest and juice of ½ a lemon

Store-cupboard essentials:
4 tablespoons Kale Crumbs
   (see page 26)
salt and pepper

Mix all the ingredients together and season with salt and pepper (for toddlers and adults).

Tip: This can be used as a dip or a spread on toast or in a sandwich. You can also experiment with different herbs and spices.

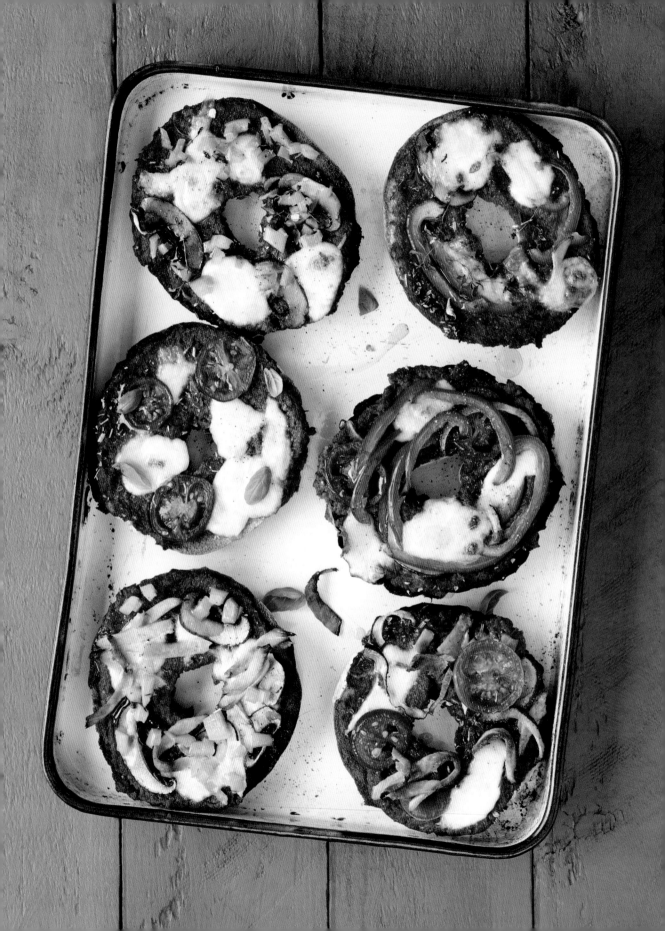

SPEEDY CHEAT'S PIZZA

Preparation time: 5 minutes
Cooking time: 12 minutes
Serves: 4

To buy:
4 white or wholegrain bagels
100g mozzarella cheese
a variety of toppings, e.g.
    mushrooms, onions, leftover
    cooked meat

Store-cupboard essentials:
1 x 400g tin tomatoes
1 teaspoon dried oregano
salt
a little extra virgin olive oil

Turn on the grill to 180°C/gas 4.

Slice the bagels in half, horizontally.

Place them on a baking tray, cut side up, and place under the grill for 5 minutes.

Blend the tomatoes with the oregano and a splash of olive oil.

Spread a thin layer of tomato sauce over the toasted bagels.

Top with cheese and your desired toppings.

Grill for 2-3 minutes, or until the cheese is golden brown.

Sprinkle the top with a little salt (for toddlers and adults).

BASIC FRITTER RECIPE

Preparation time: 5 minutes
Cooking time: 5 minutes
Makes: 12–16

Store-cupboard essentials:
1 egg
115g self-raising flour
225ml milk
salt and pepper, to taste
olive oil or butter

Mix the egg, flour and milk together in a bowl until well combined.

Add any flavour ingredients (see opposite) and seasoning (for toddlers and adults only) and stir until combined. (You may not need any additional seasoning if you are using cheese or smoked fish, or other salty ingredients.)

Heat a frying pan on a medium heat and drizzle with a little olive oil or butter.

Test to see if the pan is hot enough by dropping a small amount of batter into it . . . it should sizzle immediately.

Dollop 2 or 3 individual heaped tablespoons at a time into the pan and let each fritter cook for 1–2 minutes, until golden brown,

Flip the fritters and cook on the other side.

Serve and enjoy.

Tip: This quantity makes quite a few fritters, but the batter can be stored in the fridge for a day or two.

Pea and smoked salmon

2 slices of chopped smoked salmon
a handful of peas

Add the peas and smoked salmon to your basic fritter batter and continue with the basic method.

Tip: smoked salmon can be salty so replace with poached salmon if serving to little ones under 2 years.

Sweet potato and sweetcorn

a handful of grated sweet potato
a handful of sweetcorn

Grate the sweet potato.

Add the grated sweet potato and sweetcorn to your basic fritter batter and continue with the basic method.

4 FRITTER FLAVOURS

Courgette and Parmesan

1 grated courgette
1 handful of grated Parmesan

Place the courgette inside a kitchen towel. Squeeze all the excess liquid out of the courgette.

Add the grated courgette and Parmesan to your basic fritter batter and continue with the basic method.

Broccoli and Cheddar

4-5 broccoli florets
2 tablespoons grated Cheddar cheese

Chop the broccoli into small pieces.

Add the broccoli and Cheddar to your basic fritter batter and continue with the basic method.

Tip: You can also add Super-bean Cream (see page 90) to this recipe.

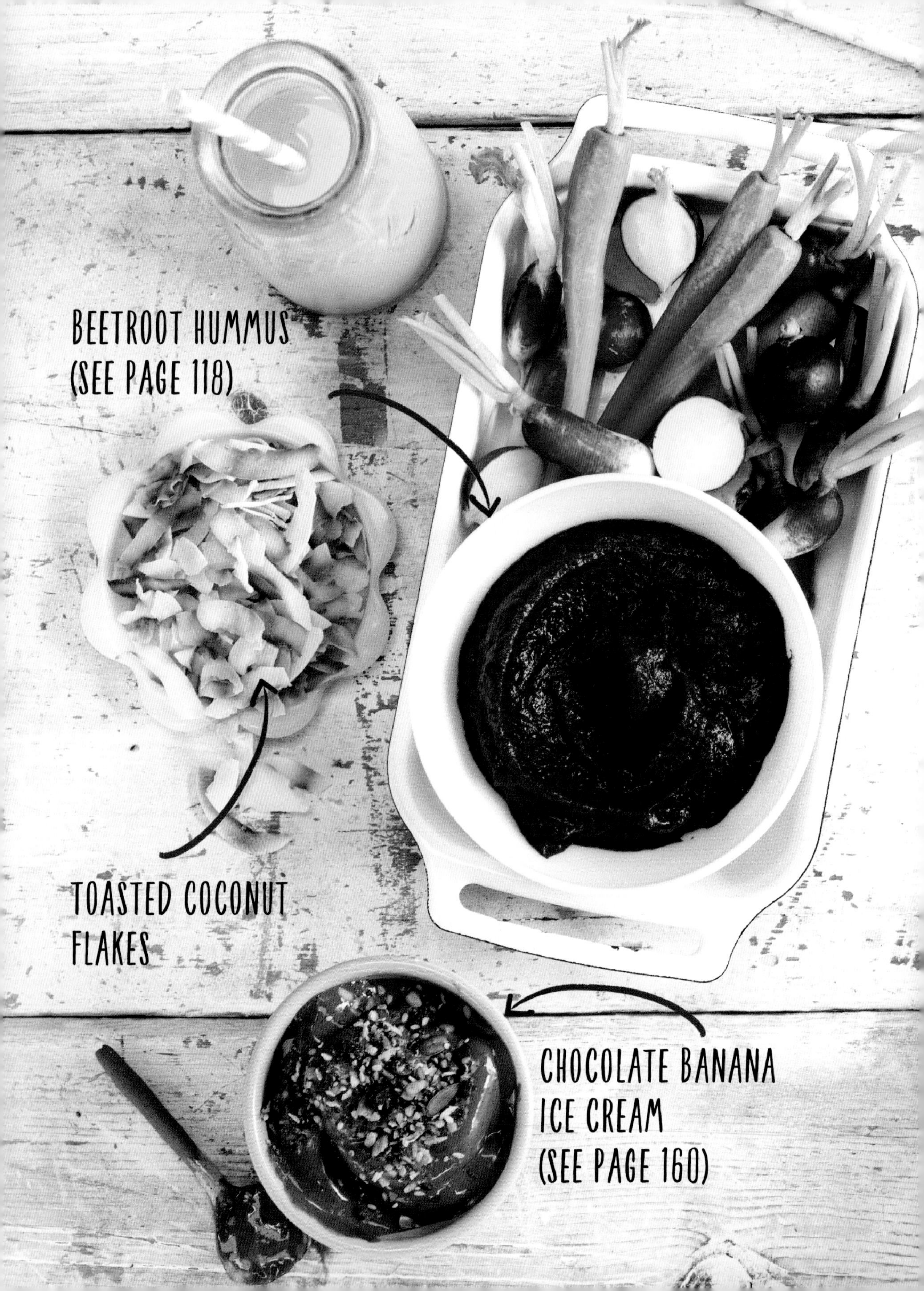

BEETROOT HUMMUS
(SEE PAGE 118)

TOASTED COCONUT
FLAKES

CHOCOLATE BANANA
ICE CREAM
(SEE PAGE 160)

TOAST CASHEW NUTS IN A PAN. ONCE GOLDEN SPRINKLE
WITH PAPRIKA. DRIZZLE WITH HONEY AND TOAST IN A PAN.
(LEAVE TO COOL COMPLETELY BEFORE SERVING).

5-MINUTE SNACKS

APPLE SANDWICH
(SEE PAGE 128)

APPLE SANDWICH

Preparation time: 5 minutes
Makes: 4

To buy:
1 red apple
1 green apple
4 tablespoons cashew
   coconut butter
   (see below)
Secret Sprinkles (see
   page 157) or a handful
   of raisins

Slice the apples widthways so you have circular slices.

Cut out the core of each apple slice using a heart or star-shaped cutter. If you don't have a cutter you can cut out a square using a knife. You should have approximately 4 slices per apple.

Spread 1 tablespoon of cashew coconut butter on each apple slice and spread it around the edges, then sandwich together two slices and coat the edges with Secret Sprinkles.

Serve and eat immediately, before the apple turns brown.

CASHEW COCONUT BUTTER

Preparation time: 2 minutes
Blending time: 2–10 minutes, depending on your food processor (this is one recipe which does require a high-speed blender to achieve a smooth consistency)
Makes: 1 small jar

To buy:
2 handfuls of
   unsweetened flaked
   coconut (approx. 30g)

Store-cupboard essentials:
2 handfuls of cashews
   (approx. 80g)
1 teaspoon vanilla extract

Place the coconut, cashews and vanilla extract in a high-speed blender or a food processor.

Blend the mixture – it will start off chunky, but with increased blending it will turn into a smooth butter. This could take anywhere between 2 and 10 minutes, depending on how powerful your food processor is. Be careful not to overheat your machine. (Tip: You can add a little melted coconut oil to the mixture to loosen it to your preference.)

Store in the fridge in an airtight container for up to 2 months.

Tips: Feel free to use any other type of nut butter, like almond or peanut, and to sprinkle with chocolate chips or another dried fruit like cranberries.

Soak the apple slices in water and the juice of a lemon to stop them turning brown.

HONEY CINNAMON ROASTED CHICKPEAS

Preparation time: 15 minutes
Cooking time: 60–90 minutes
Serves: many!

Store-cupboard essentials:

4 teaspoons olive oil
2 x 400g tins of chickpeas
2 teaspoons ground cinnamon
2 tablespoons honey (avoid serving
  to baby under 1 year)

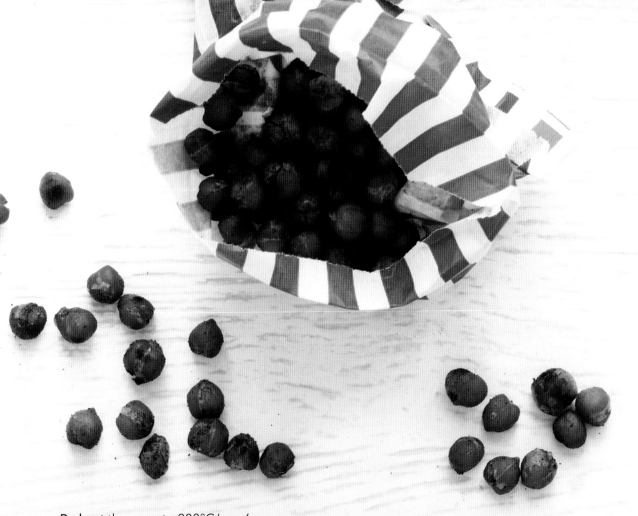

Preheat the oven to 200°C/gas 6.

Drain the chickpeas and rinse them under cold water. Dry them on a paper towel.

Whisk the oil and cinnamon together in a small bowl. Add the chickpeas to the bowl and stir until they are all evenly coated.

Spread out the chickpeas on a large baking sheet.

Bake for 60-90 minutes, or until the chickpeas are crunchy and no longer soft in the middle.

Place the hot, roasted chickpeas in a small bowl and coat evenly with honey.

Spread the chickpeas back on the baking sheet and allow to dry.

Store in an airtight container at room temperature.

Chop these up into small pieces for babies and toddlers.

IDEAS FOR PARTY SNACKS

These are some of our favourite party snacks.

BUCKWHEAT
JAMMY DODGERS
(SEE PAGE 143)

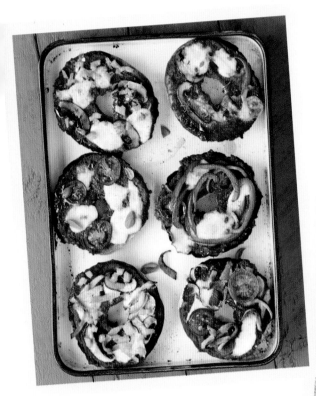

SPEEDY CHEAT'S
PIZZA (SEE PAGE 123)

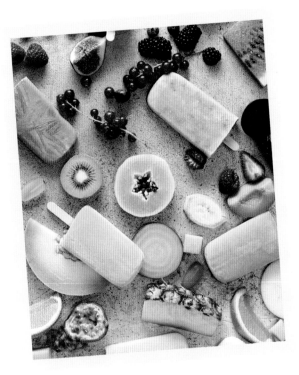

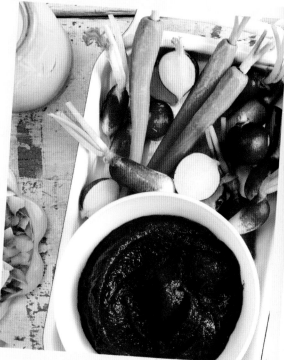

BEETROOT HUMMUS
(SEE PAGE 118)

FROZEN FRUIT LOLLIES
(SEE PAGE 145)

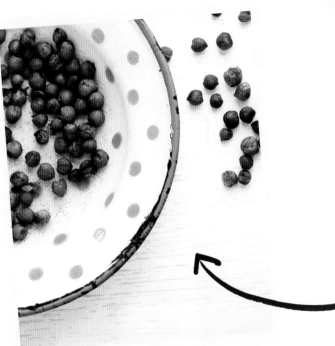

CRISPY CHICKEN
TENDERS (SEE PAGE 207)

HONEY CINNAMON
ROASTED CHICKPEAS
(SEE PAGE 130)

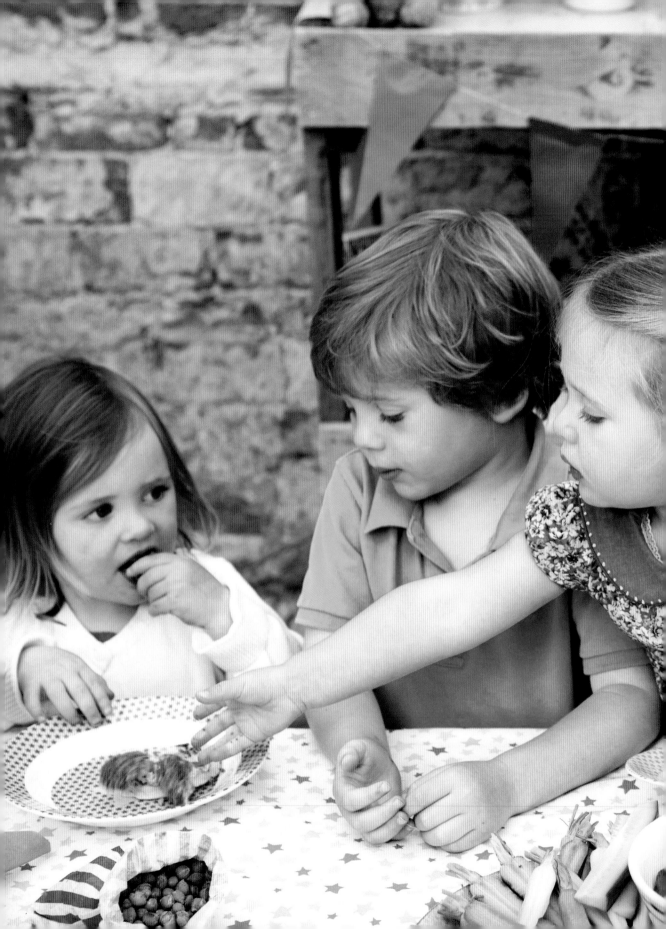

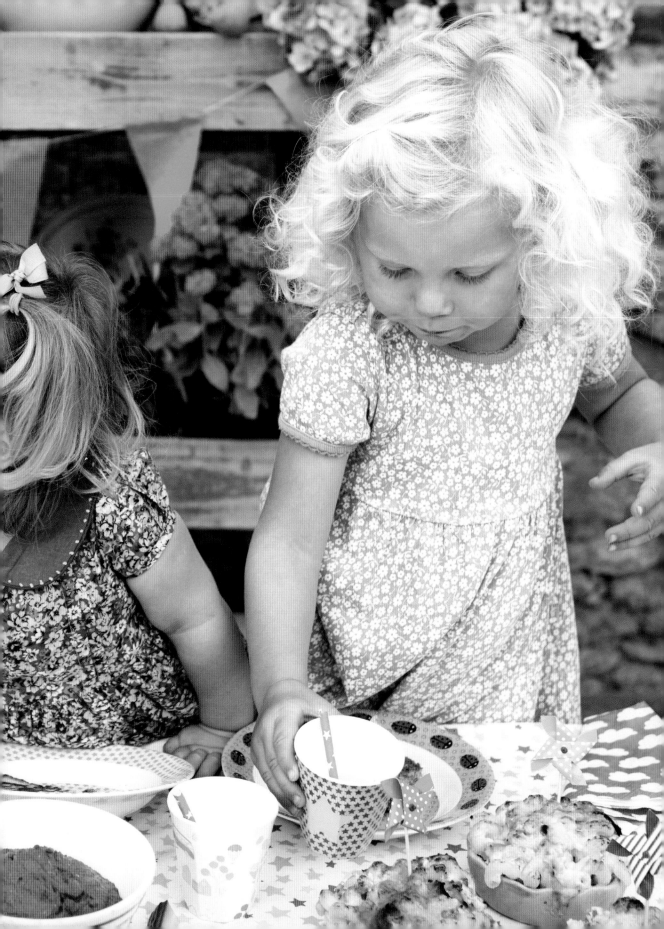

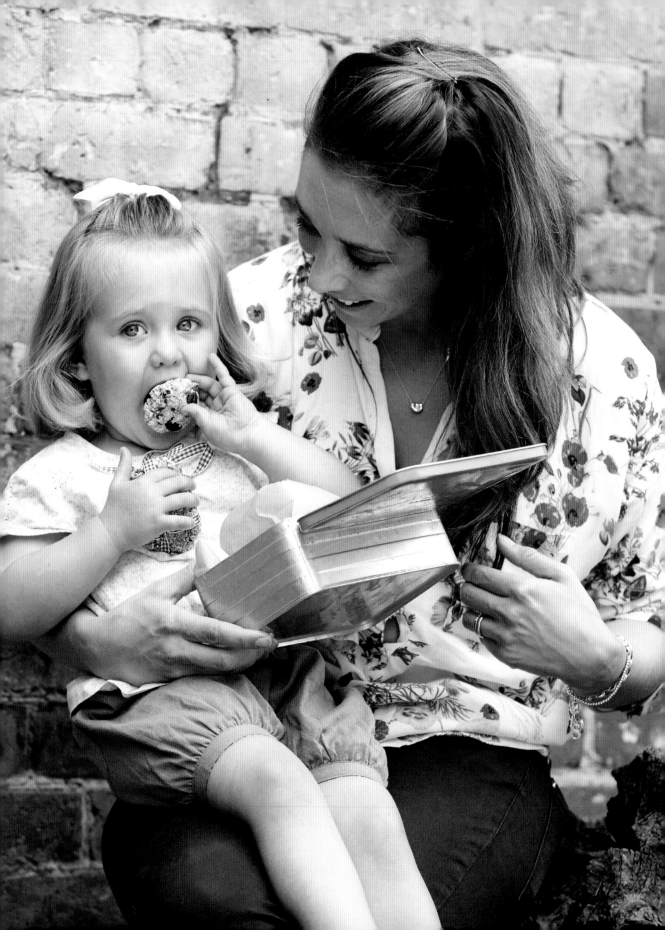

OATY BANANA BISCUITS

These can be made without the honey or maple syrup if you're conscious of sugar intake.

Preparation time: 10 minutes
Cooking time: 10–12 minutes
Makes: 12–16

To buy:
1 large ripe banana

Store-cupboard essentials:
100g oats
2 tablespoons raisins
1 tablespoon maple syrup or honey
(avoid honey if serving to baby
under 1 year)
2 tablespoons chopped nuts,
seeds or chocolate (almonds,
walnuts, peanuts, pistachios,
choc chips, etc.)

Preheat the oven to 160°C/gas 3.

Place some baking parchment on a baking tray.

Blitz the oats in the pot attachment of your stick blender for a couple of minutes until they are of a fine consistency.

Mash the banana in a bowl and add the raisins and maple syrup.

Add the oats and 2 tablespoons of your choice of crunch to the banana mix.

Spoon a heaped tablespoon of the mixture on to the baking parchment.

Bake for 10-12 minutes, until the cookies are just getting crisp on the outside but are still soft in the middle. The cookies are best eaten the day they are made, but can also be stored in an airtight biscuit tin for up to 2 days.

Tip: If you don't have raisins to hand, you can use any other chopped dried fruit you might have.

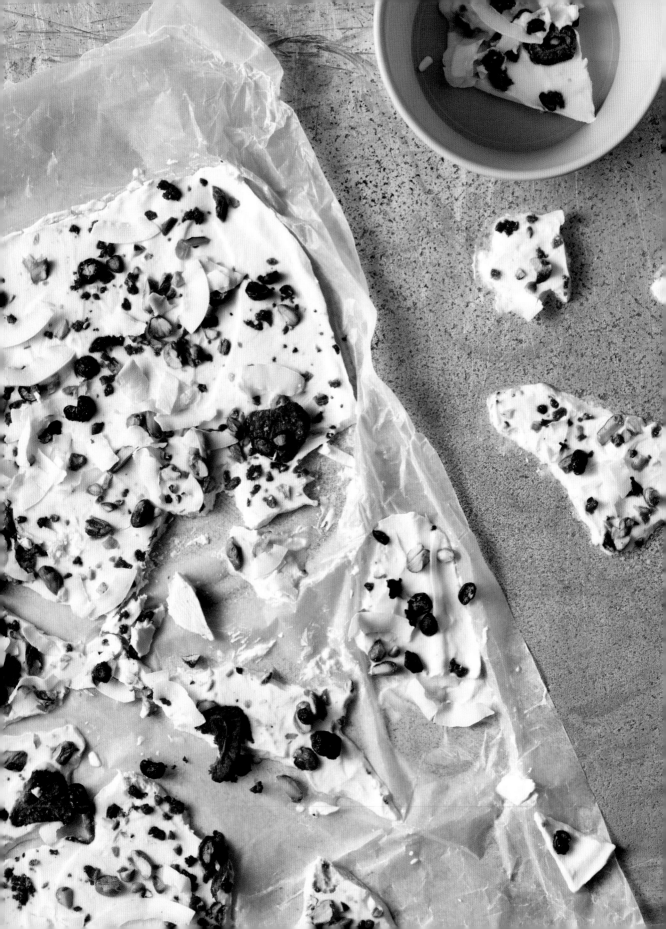

FROZEN YOGHURT BERRY BARK

Preparation time: 10 minutes
Freezing time: overnight
Serves: many

To buy:
150g full-fat thick Greek yoghurt
2 tablespoons freeze-dried or fresh
  strawberries

Store-cupboard essentials:
2 tablespoons chopped pistachios,
  or other nut of your choice

Line a baking tray or small freezer-safe pan with greaseproof paper.

Roughly chop the pistachios.

Spread the yoghurt thinly, about 1cm thick, on the greaseproof paper.

Sprinkle the pistachios and strawberries evenly over the yoghurt.

Freeze uncovered overnight.

Remove from the baking sheet once frozen.

Break into small pieces and serve immediately as it defrosts quickly.

Store extra pieces in a freezer-safe container.

Tip: Wrap baking paper around the pieces of bark when serving, to help little ones eat it (it can be cold to hold and melts quickly).

SMOOTHIES: FORMULA

Simply add one ingredient from each section to make your perfect combo.
As a general guide, we use a handful of each ingredient and just a sprinkle of
flavour before whizzing. Then we adjust the quantities to suit our tastebuds . . .
(e.g. more fruit for extra sweetness or more cream for some added luxury).

THE FRUIT +

e.g. pineapple
mango
berries
banana
kiwi

THE CREAM +

e.g. milk
yoghurt
coconut milk
single cream
avocado

THE HIDDEN +

e.g. Kale Crumbs
(see page 26)
spinach
Beetroot Blitz
(see page 91)

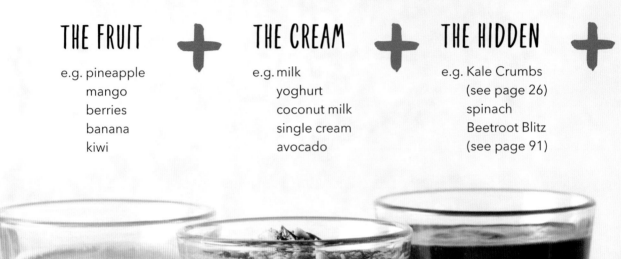

Here are some
of our favourite
combinations:

GROOVY GREEN

Apple
Kiwi
Kale Crumbs
Greek yoghurt
Ground almonds

SUMMER SHERBET

Raspberries/strawberries
Peach
Greek yoghurt
Porridge oats
Honey

THE CRUNCH

e.g. oats
    ground nuts
    Secret Sprinkles
    (see page 157)
    seeds (flax, chia,
    sunflower)
    coconut flakes

+

THE FLAVOUR

e.g. cinnamon
    cocoa powder
    ginger
    mint
    honey (not for
    baby under
    1 year)

=

THE WHIZ

Blend and loosen
to desired
consistency with
water or milk

CARIBBEAN COCONUT

Banana
Pineapple
Coconut milk
Desiccated coconut (optional)

MOODY BLUES

Avocado
Blueberries
Coconut milk
Seeds

COCOA OATS

Avocado
Cocoa powder
Banana
Milk (regular, almond
or hazelnut)
Porridge oats

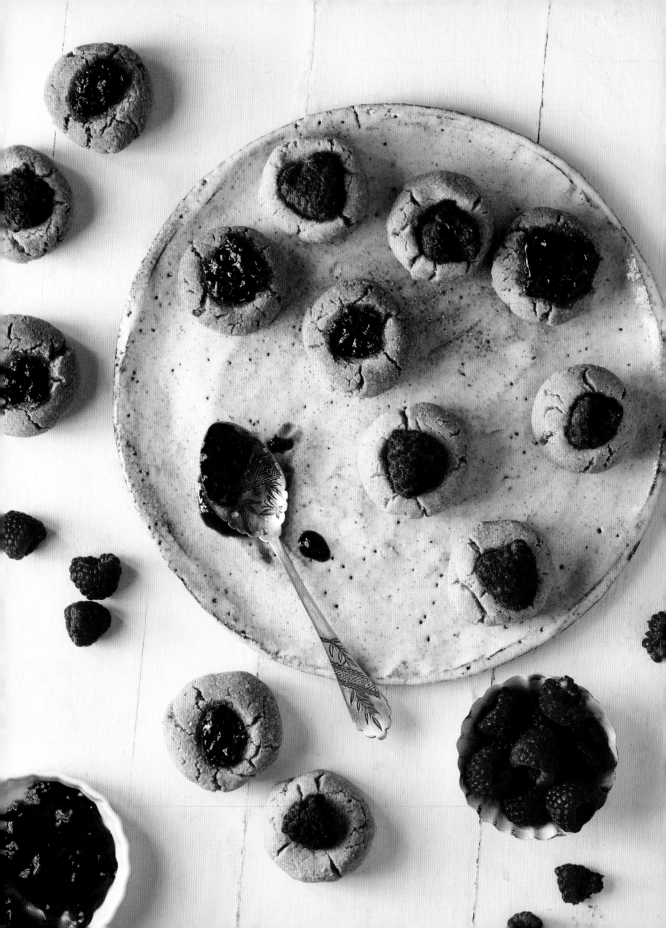

BUCKWHEAT JAMMY DODGERS

Preparation time: 15 minutes
Cooking time: 15 minutes
Makes: 24

To buy:
300g buckwheat or plain flour
180g ground almonds
for the filling: either fresh
   raspberries or raspberry jam

Store-cupboard essentials:
¼ teaspoon salt (omit if serving to baby)
1 teaspoon ground cinnamon
160ml maple syrup (or 8 tablespoons)
125ml olive oil

Preheat the oven to 180°C/gas 4.

Line two baking trays with parchment paper.

Mix all the ingredients together in a large bowl, except the raspberries
or jam.

Take heaped tablespoons of the mixture, roll into balls, and place
on the prepared trays leaving a 2cm space between them.

Press your thumb into the centre of each ball and place a raspberry
(or a teaspoon of jam) in the centre.

Bake for 15 minutes, until golden.

Leave to cool on a cooling rack.

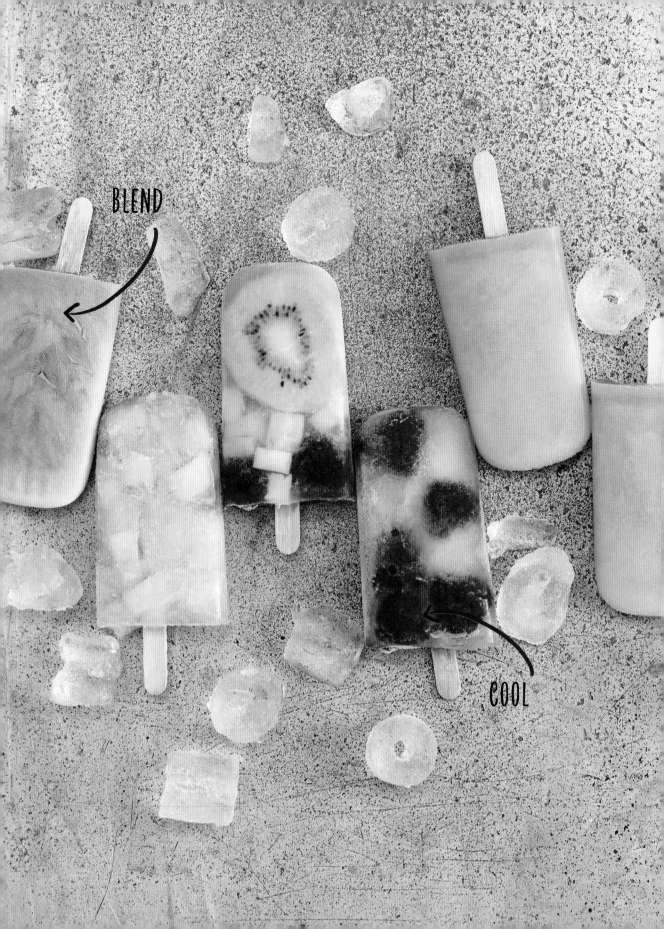

BLEND

COOL

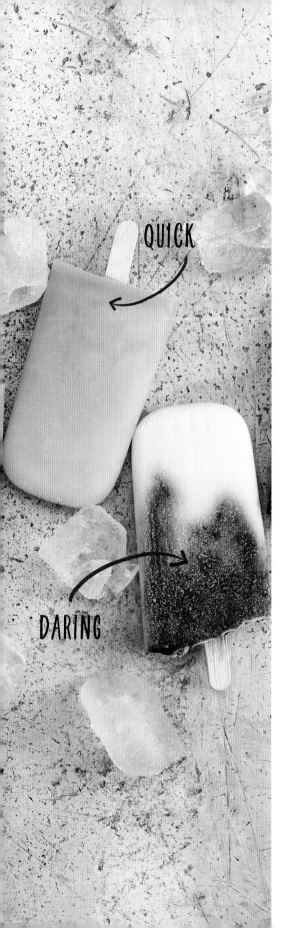

FRUIT LOLLIES

BLEND

Freeze a smoothie in a lolly mould (see pages 140-41 for smoothie combos).

COOL

Place fruit chunks in a lolly mould and cover with elderflower water, then freeze.

QUICK

Freeze fruit juice (e.g. orange, grapefruit, apple) in a lolly mould. Simple!

DARING

Fill a lolly mould three-quarters of the way up with thick full-fat Greek yoghurt, then add fruit purée up to the top and use a lolly stick to push the purée into the yoghurt to create a marbled effect. Freeze until solid.

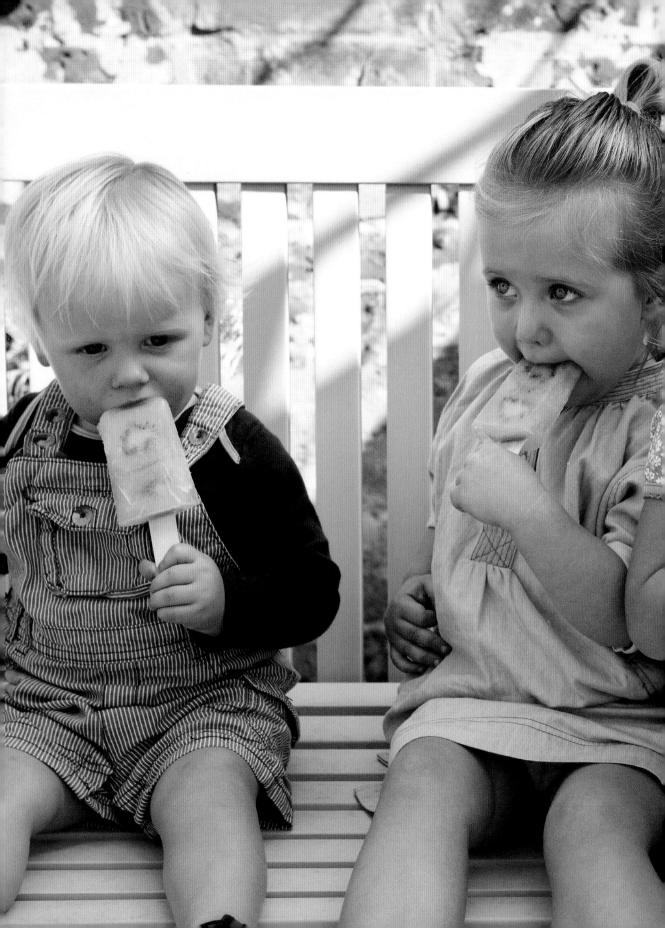

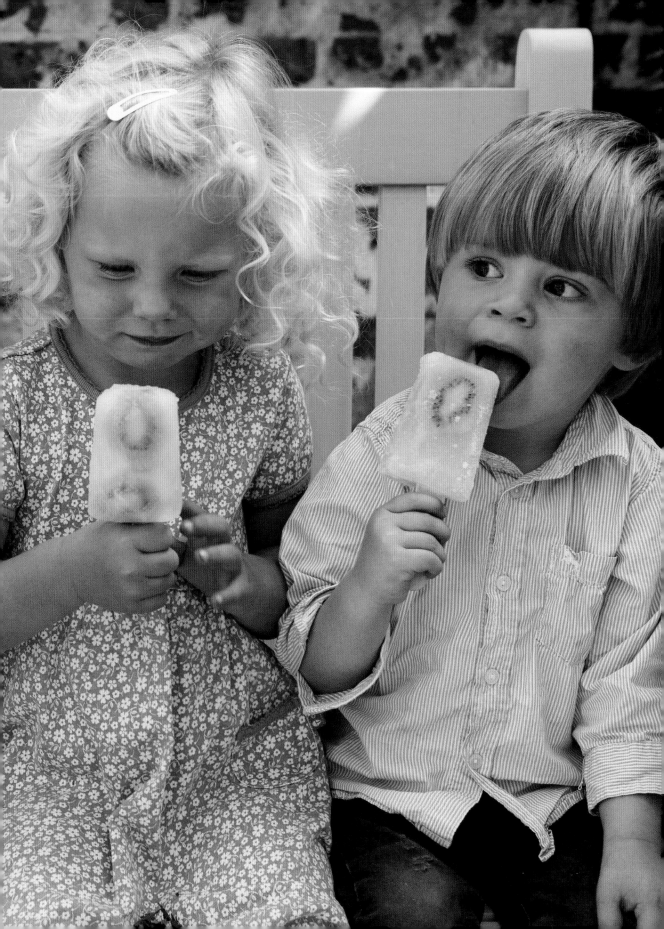

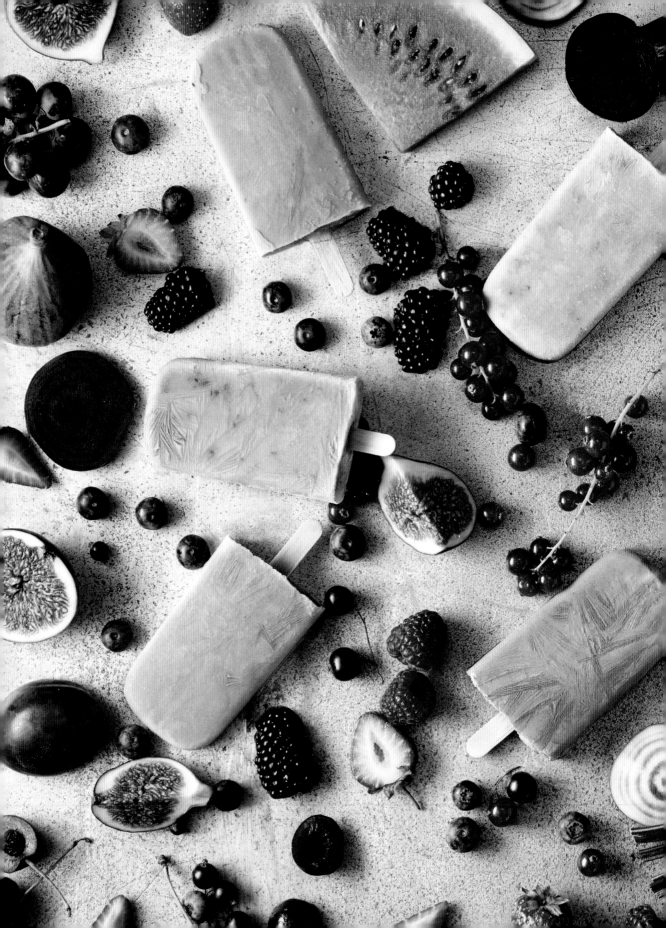

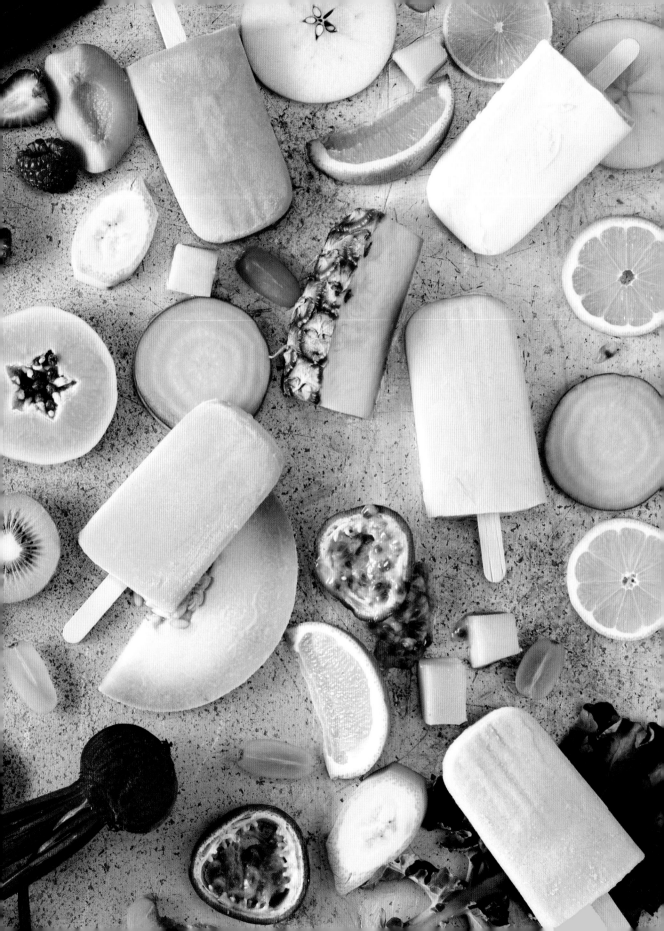

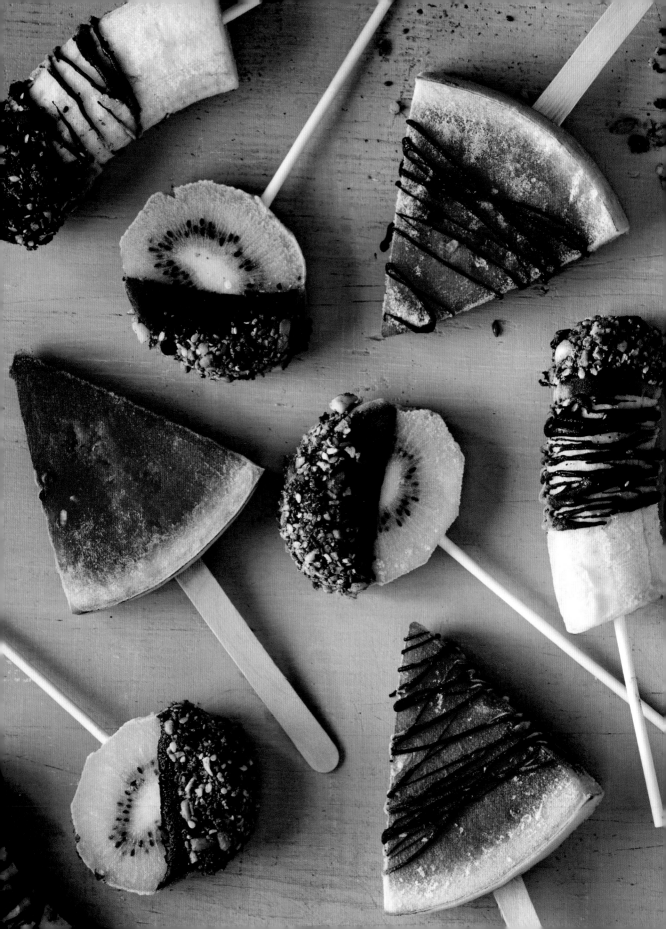

FROZEN FRUIT LOLLIPOPS

Preparation time: 5–15 minutes
Freezing time: 2–3 hours

To buy:
watermelon, cut into triangles
   with skin left on
kiwi, peeled and cut into
   round discs
bananas, peeled
wooden lolly sticks

Optional:
melted chocolate
Secret Sprinkles (see page 157)

Cut a small slit in the skin of the watermelon, the disc of kiwi and the bottom of a banana, then place a lolly stick in the slit and freeze.

Optional: once the fruit is frozen, for an extra treat you can dip it in melted chocolate, sprinkle with our Secret Sprinkles, then freeze for a further 5–10 minutes.

Tip: You can also dip the fruit in Greek yoghurt for a healthier topping.

Have fun experimenting with other fruits e.g. mango, peaches or pineapple.

BUCKWHEAT GINGER NUTS

Preparation time: 15 minutes
Cooking time: 15 minutes
Makes: 24

To buy:
300g buckwheat or plain flour
180g ground almonds

Store-cupboard essentials:
¼ teaspoon salt (omit if serving to baby)
160ml maple syrup (or 8 tablespoons)
125ml olive oil
1 teaspoon fresh or ground ginger
for the filling: 28 whole almonds

Preheat your oven to 180°C/gas 4.

Line two baking trays with baking paper.

Mix all the ingredients together in a large bowl, except the whole almonds.

Take heaped tablespoons of the mixture, roll into balls, and place them on the prepared trays, leaving a 2cm space between them.

Press your thumb into the centre of each ball and place a whole almond in the centre.

Bake for 15 minutes, until golden.

Leave to cool on a cooling rack.

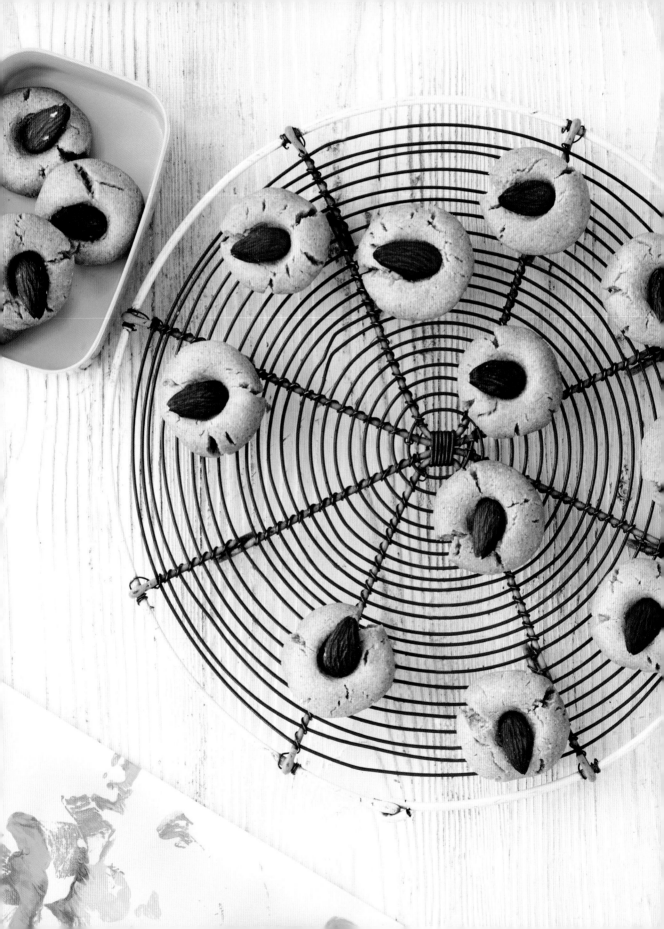

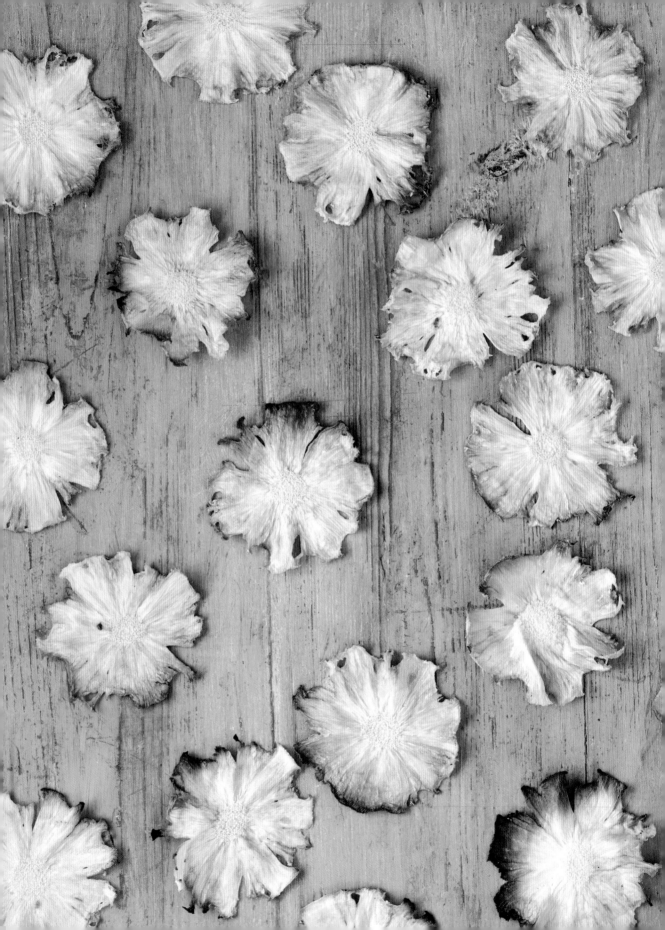

PINEAPPLE CHIPS

Preparation time: 15 minutes
Cooking time: 40 minutes
Cooling time: overnight
Serves: 2–4

To buy:

1 pineapple

Preheat oven to 120°C/gas ½.

Cut both ends off the pineapple and remove the skin.

Scoop with a strawberry corer or melon baller (use a knife if you don't have either) to remove random round pieces of pineapple, keeping the pineapple whole. (This will help to create the flower effect but is not necessary for taste.)

Keep the round pieces of pineapple for a separate snack.

Cut wafer thin discs of pineapple, using a mandolin or sharp knife to get them as thin as possible.

Place on a baking tray lined with parchment paper and bake in the oven for 20 minutes.

Remove from the oven after the initial 20 minutes and turn them over. Then bake for a further 20 minutes.

Turn the oven off and leave in the oven overnight, so that they cool and crisp up.

Tip: These can be eaten immediately, but if you want them to be crispy leave them in the turned-off oven overnight.

USE ANY COMBINATION
OF NUTS/SEEDS/DRIED
FRUITS YOU LIKE.

SECRET SPRINKLES

Preparation time: 5 minutes
Makes: 1 jar

To buy:

1 tablespoon dried cranberries
1 tablespoon raisins
1 tablespoon dried apricots
1 tablespoon unsweetened
  desiccated coconut
1 tablespoon pistachios
1 tablespoon almonds
1 tablespoon pecans

Store-cupboard essentials:

1 teaspoon ground cinnamon
1 tablespoon sunflower seeds
1 tablespoon flax seeds
1 tablespoon chia seeds
1 tablespoon sesame seeds
1 tablespoon pumpkin seeds
1 tablespoon cocoa nibs

Place all the ingredients in your blender pot attachment and blitz until roughly chopped.

Sprinkle over yoghurt, ice cream, smoothies, soups, cereal, etc.

Store in an airtight container – the sprinkles keep for a few weeks.

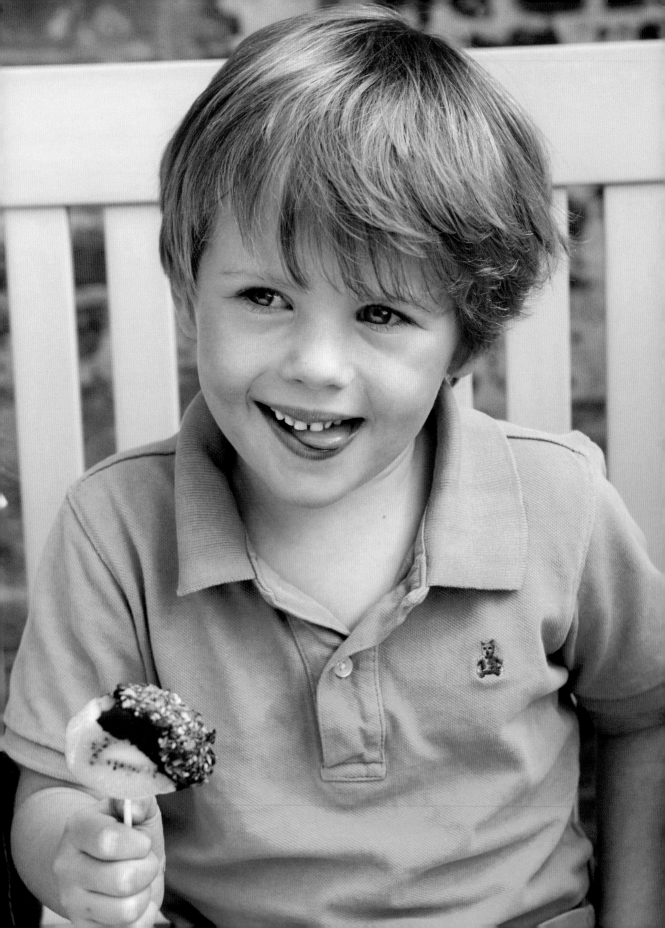

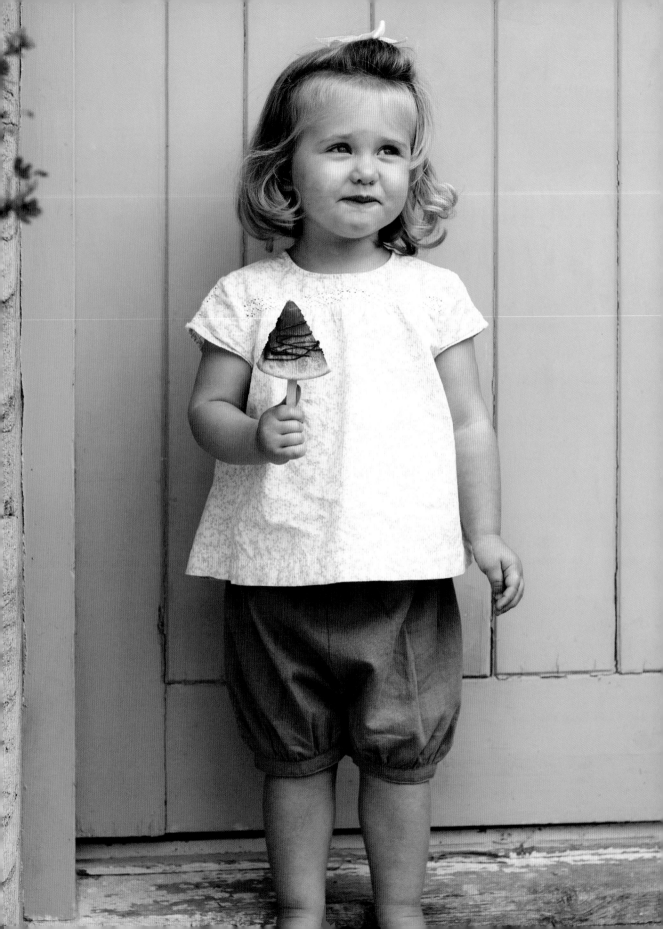

CHOCOLATE BANANA ICE CREAM

Preparation time: 2 minutes
Serves: 1–2

To buy:
2 bananas, frozen
2 teaspoons cocoa powder

Store-cupboard essentials:
a splash of milk
2 teaspoons maple syrup
    or honey (optional) (avoid honey
    if serving to baby under 1 year)

Place all the ingredients in a blender and blitz until smooth (you can use a stick blender too).

Serve immediately.

Tip: We love to scatter Secret Sprinkles (see page 157) on top of this ice cream.

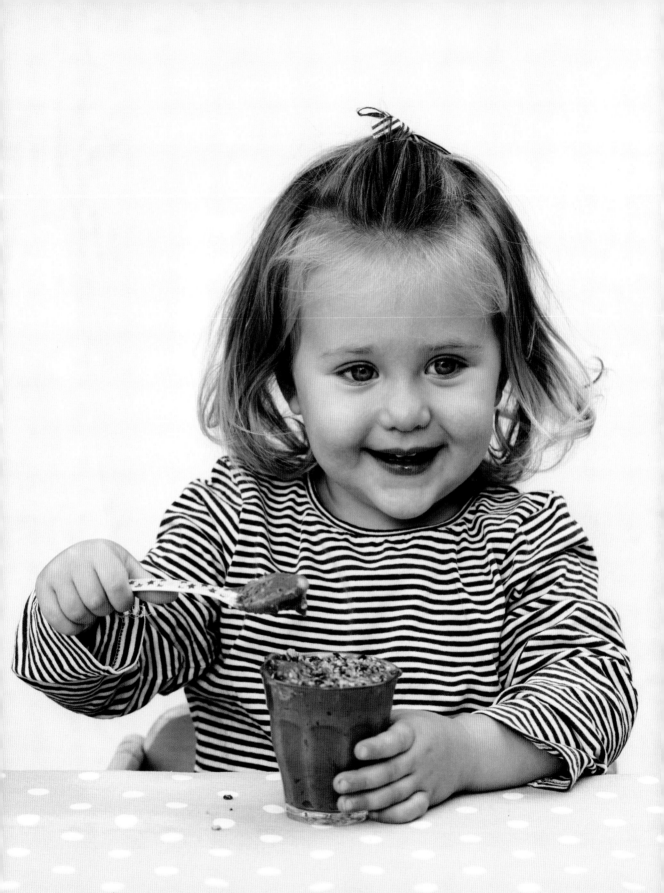

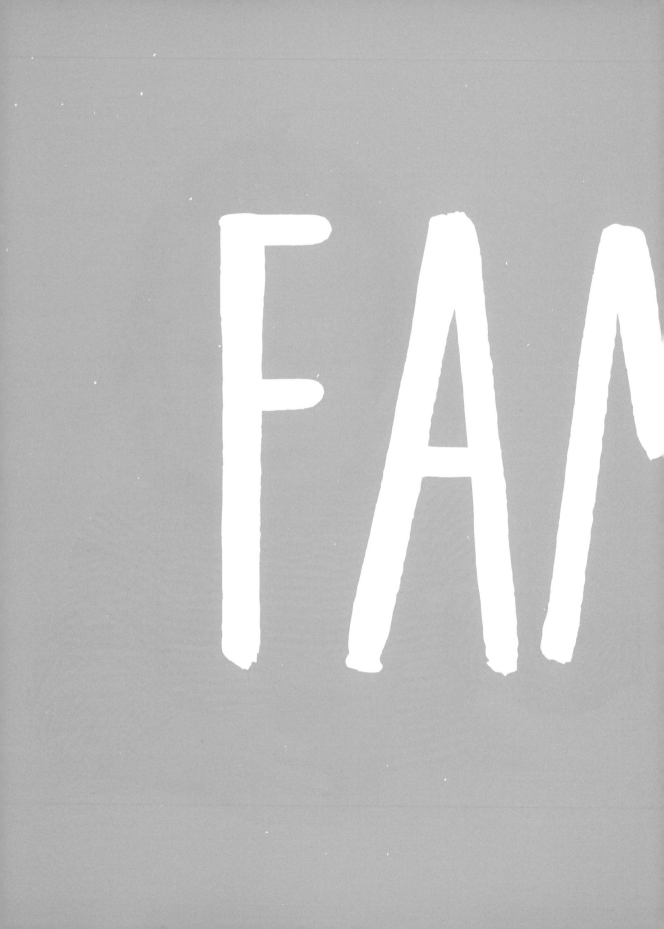

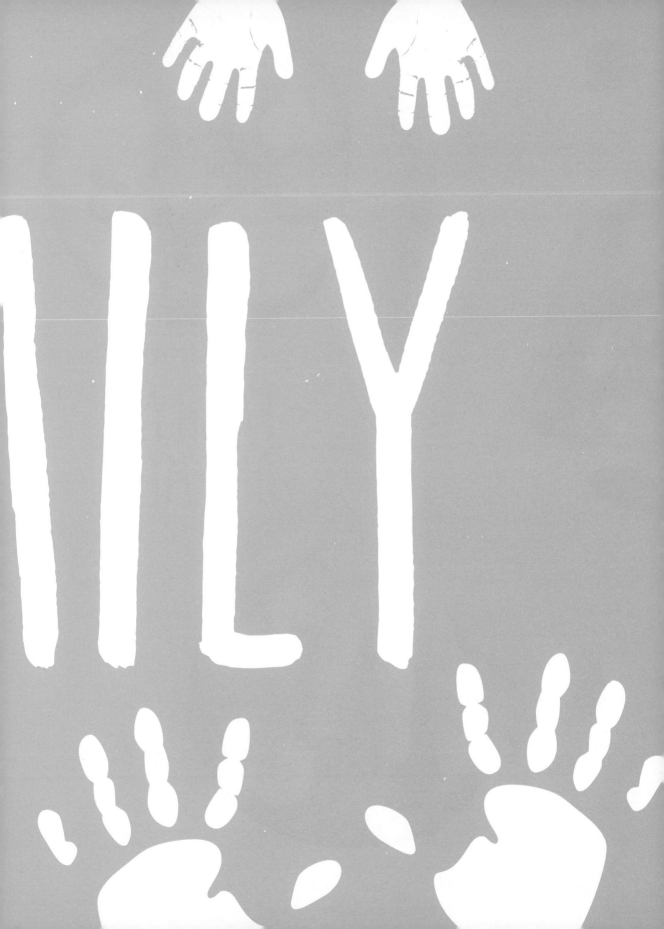

FAMILY:
ONE MEAL

One thing I'm passionate about is the importance of involving children in the kitchen as early as possible; that's how my sisters and I were brought up, and it's how we learnt the importance of eating well and cooking the basics. Our family's philosophy is that *la tavola* (the kitchen table) is the most sacred place in the house – it's the place we eat, cook, socialize and interact, the heartbeat of the family. And this is something we want to pass down to our children.

My mum has always advised that this 'food education' starts from the very beginning – from the moment a child is born. Babies, toddlers and kids will absorb a huge amount just by being in the same space as you while you cook . . . sounds, smells and tastes. Think how quickly a baby starts to copy your actions and sounds . . . so let them watch you while you prepare.

Find me a child who doesn't enjoy being involved in the kitchen – getting messy, of course! A place full of textures, tastes and smells... the ultimate playgroup, right in your own home.

Similarly, toddlers absolutely love being involved – try to get them to do any cooking preparation with you, as even the simplest of jobs can keep them entertained. Fiamma loves to pick basil leaves for me to make her pesto. Older kids can have fun activities linked to food (ask them to draw your shopping list and follow you around the supermarket), or you can simply get them used to helping you lay the table.

I believe the more involved your children feel in the kitchen, the more they will want to learn and explore new tastes as they grow. Food and family are intrinsically linked for Italians and are at the heart of eating well. Whether you are from a small or large family, everyone can create a family unit or friendship group that unites and socializes around food and *la tavola*. Ditch the 'kids' meals' and make it your goal to feed your family one meal together. This is what this chapter, and ultimately the whole book, is about.

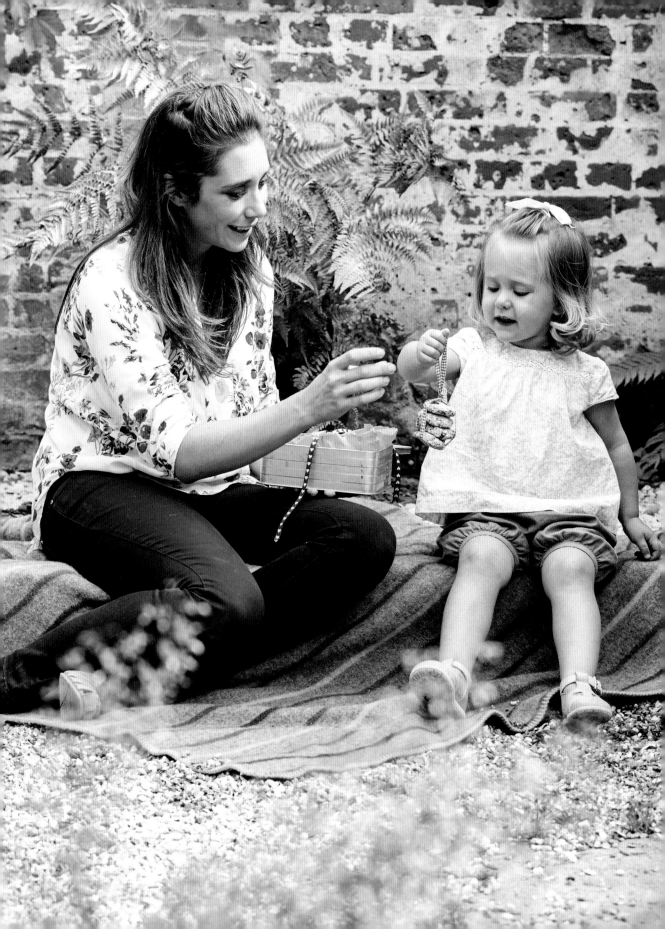

SECRETS OF SUCCESS

Be realistic.

Don't over-complicate your cooking and be realistic about what is achievable and when. For example, weekdays are always hectic for me; if it's the same for you, this is the time to dive into those freezer essentials or rustle up that cheat's pasta sauce. Don't try to be innovative on these nights or give yourself unnecessary pressure, even if you think you have the time. Keep the experiments to the weekends, when there is more time available. And don't feel guilty if you do have the odd cheat's takeaway . . . Why not? It's not about being perfect, but about trying to do the best you can.

Make mealtimes a social occasion.

Try to get your family or friendship group to eat together, as a unit, as often as possible. This is the Italian way, and there are huge benefits in creating a sense of unity once a day. I'm certainly not perfect, and we all have challenges, whether it's long working hours or the deflated feeling of trying to cook a nice meal that ends with the kids arguing and eating in deathly silence. My advice here is to keep mealtimes simple and lighthearted . . . Don't try to attempt something complex if you don't have the time. Hopefully the recipes in this book can help. However, even if it only happens at a weekend, where possible try to get into the habit of sitting together and making your mealtimes a relaxed and social occasion. And if it fails, try again another time.

Variety.

Try to mix up your cooking. It's about varying not just your ingredients, but also the way you cook them. Try not to fall into the trap of cooking your food the same way each time . . . If you like roast veg, try pan-frying vegetables some days, grating them into salads or fritters on others, grilling them, making soups, serving them as finger foods with dips or making a new pesto sauce.

Try not to stress.

Keeping a relaxed attitude at mealtimes will honestly have a positive impact. Anxiety that your baby/toddler hasn't eaten enough food or the right food will just stress everyone out. Kids will eat if they are hungry. If they don't feel like it now, try another time. Keep the environment relaxed and social. Equally, preparing food shouldn't be stressful either. If it's not in your nature to experiment with foods, take it a step at a time. Pick a day of the week where you'll try new things, or invite friends round and take it in turns to cook for each other (one night you're busy, but then you get two or three nights off in return!). Happy mum, happy family!

Buy the best you can afford.

Cooking fresh can be expensive, so just buy the best you can afford. Buying in bulk, certainly if you are planning to do batch cooking for your freezer, can often be the best way to keep costs down.

Keep it pure.

Unprocessed, full-fat foods are the best, in my opinion. Processed foods which claim to be low in fat or free from added sugar will often have lots of hidden nasties in them. If you want to eat butter, eat the most natural, unprocessed and full-fat version (just maybe have a small portion).

Flexibility.

Remember, you don't have to follow recipes religiously. With many savoury recipes you can often swap in different veggies or cheeses or meats and create different versions of your favourite dishes. So if you especially love a recipe, see if you can mix it up with different herbs/veg/other ingredients.

The banned ingredient.

Try not to ban foods or deny a child who is curious. Wanting a treat is perfectly natural, so allow your kids to have the odd biscuit or other treat – banning them will make them all the more desirable.

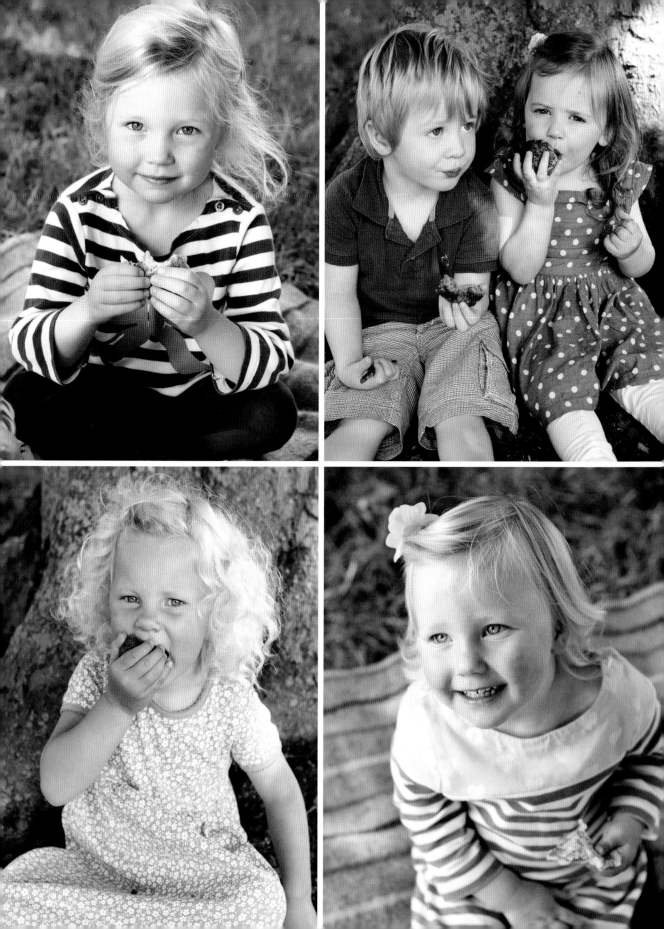

HOW I DID IT

Here are some tips that
really worked for me:

Fun with food.

My eldest loves to pretend to cook. She makes cakes using sand at the beach and pizzas using leaves and grass in the garden. My youngest enjoys stirring pasta shapes in different saucepans in the kitchen. Older kids love designing menus for dinnertime or drawing the ingredients on a shopping list. Encourage older kids to grow herbs from seed, and get the younger ones to smell, touch and taste different herbs.

Get the kids involved.

Get the kids involved in any way you can when preparing food. My 2-year-old loves helping me chop, with a blunt kids' knife of course (it requires her full concentration, which occupies her for ages!). Getting them to mix and mash things is also a good idea.

No TV at mealtimes.

Growing up in an Italian family, mealtimes were rituals. We used to beg our father to let us watch our favourite TV show for special treats, but he never caved in. Not once. We would initially moan and groan, but in the end we gave in and knew it wasn't worth the argument. Looking back now, as a parent myself, I can see the value in keeping these moments TV-free. Mealtimes give you the chance to connect as a family and interact, so try to keep these times sacred. Be strict about it – your kids will pick up all sorts (like table manners) from simply watching you interact.

Controversial.

In my big family, babies are always passed around from one family member to another, allowing me very little chance to fully control what went into my babies' mouths. After 6 months, both Fiamma and Serafina had their fingers dipped into tiramisu (despite raw eggs being a massive no for babies), wine, coffee and sugar bowls. Like I said – controversial! I grew up eating around a dinner table where wine was always part of every meal and we were encouraged to taste everything the adults had – from scallops to tripe. Our nonna always said, never refuse a baby if it is keen to explore a new taste. Obviously don't give them a whole glass of wine (!); however, a tiny dip in the glass with their finger is not going to harm them, and actually will encourage them to be curious about their food. This is something you need to decide as a parent, but I often think complete refusal of something makes kids want it more later on.

Plan.
Where possible, try to plan ahead. Find a time in the week when you can do some batch cooking and make it enjoyable – I like doing this on a Sunday evening, as I usually get my husband to do bath and bedtimes. I crack open a bottle of wine, plug in some tunes and busy myself for a couple of hours in the kitchen. Those 2 hours will often set me up for at least a week of speedy freezer meals.

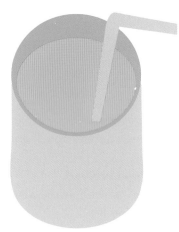

MIX UP YOUR STYLE OF COOKING TO KEEP YOUR KIDS USED TO VARIETY.

Try to make sure that each week you are
feeding them mixed styles of cooking . . .

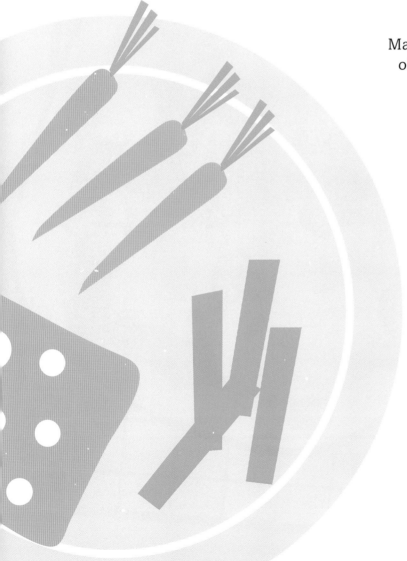

FINGER FOODS.

Finger foods or separated foods on a plate. Often easiest for lunch, snacks and picnics (e.g. sandwiches, cheese, ham, chicken nuggets, etc.).

BLITZED SOUPS.

Make sure you also give a range of blitzed foods, and blended or liquidy textures (soups, smoothies, etc.).

COMBO MEALS.

Make sure they have a selection of combo meals too, i.e. ones with mixed textures and lumps (stews with rice, casseroles with chunky veg, etc.).

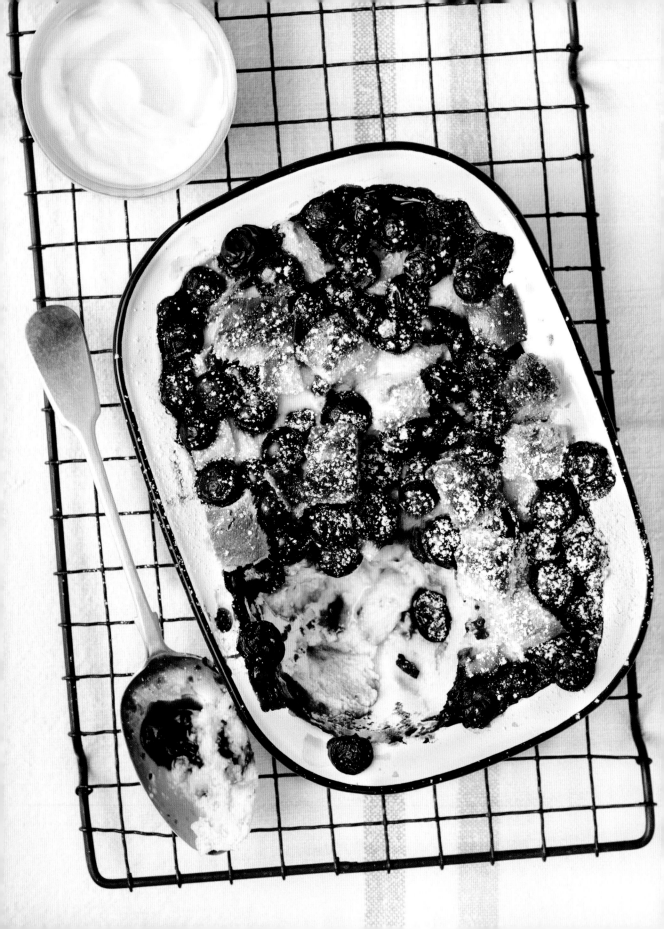

BERRY BAKE

Preparation time: 15 minutes
Cooking time: 35–40 minutes
Serves: 6–8

To buy:
3-4 slices of brioche or any sweet
    bread (150g)
4 handfuls of blueberries (200g)
1 tub of cream cheese (180g)
icing sugar, to sprinkle on top
    (optional)

Store-cupboard essentials:
4 tablespoons honey (or maple
    syrup if serving to baby under
    1 year)
2 eggs
1 teaspoon vanilla extract
225ml milk

Preheat the oven to 180°C/gas 4.

Cut the brioche into 2cm cubes and place in a greased 23cm square ovenproof dish.

Sprinkle with the berries.

Beat the cream cheese, honey, eggs and vanilla extract in a medium bowl using an electric mixer until well blended.

Slowly add the milk while continuing to whisk.

Pour the milk mixture over the brioche and blueberries and leave to soak in for 20 minutes, or overnight in the fridge.

Bake for 35-40 minutes, or until set in the centre and golden brown.

Cover with foil for the last 5-10 minutes if the surface is getting too brown.

Serve warm, sprinkled with icing sugar.

Tip: Instead of using brioche you could also make this with croissants and use different fruits.

BASIC PANCAKE MIX

Preparation time: 5 minutes
Cooking time: 5 minutes
Serves: 3–4

Store-cupboard essentials:
100g plain flour
100ml whole milk
1 egg
oil or butter, for frying

Mix all the ingredients together in a bowl until well combined.

Add any flavour ingredient (see below) and mix well.

Heat a non-stick frying pan on a medium heat.

Drizzle a little olive oil or butter into the pan and let it heat up.

Dollop a tablespoon of batter at a time into the pan and cook for
2-3 minutes on each side, until golden brown.

Flavour ingredients:

Add 1 tablespoon Beetroot Blitz (see page 91) to make pink pancakes.

Add 1 tablespoon puréed sweet potato to make orange pancakes.

Substitute the milk with coconut milk and add 1 tablespoon unsweetened
desiccated coconut for coconut pancakes.

Cut an apple or pear into discs, dip into the batter and fry for a fruity fritter.

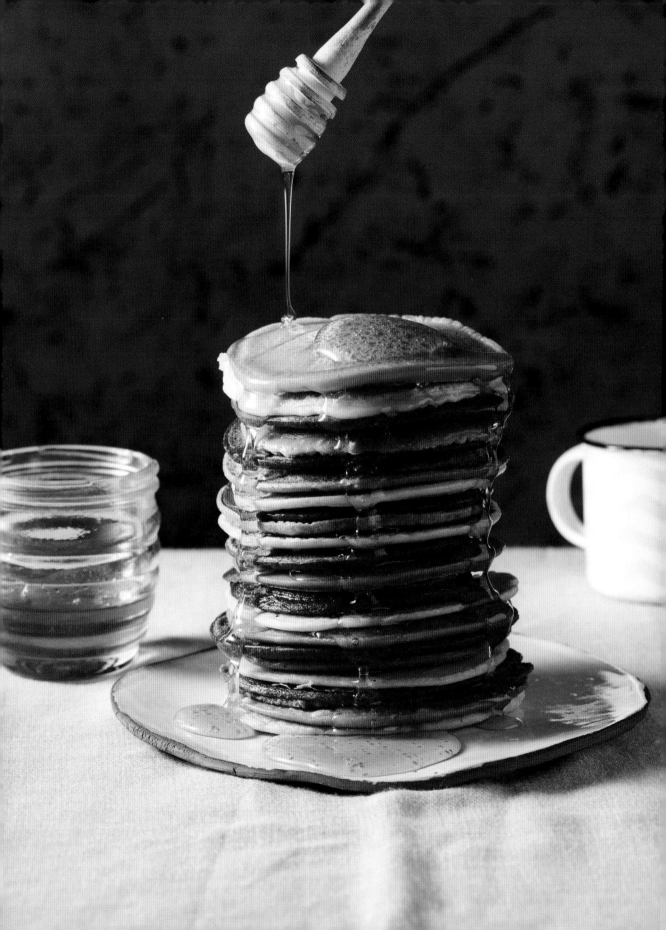

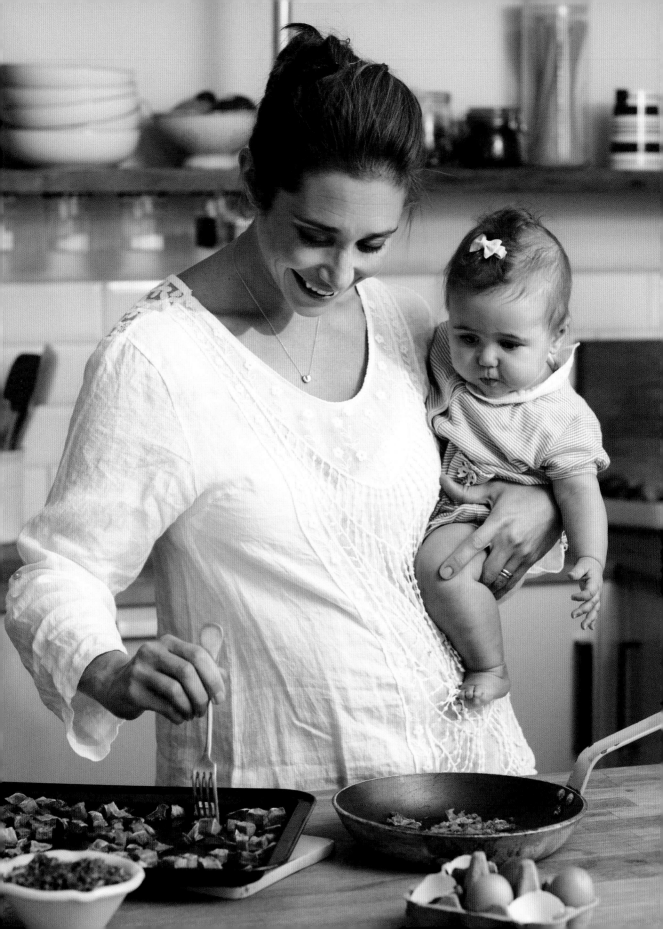

HEALTHY FAMILY FRITTATA

Preparation time: 10 minutes
Cooking time: 20–30 minutes
Serves: 3–4

To buy:
a handful of leftover roasted veg (sweet
  potato, parsnip, butternut squash)

Store-cupboard essentials:
2 eggs
1 tablespoon Kale Crumbs
  (see page 26)
salt and pepper, to taste

Mash your roasted vegetables with a fork and place in a non-stick frying pan.

Add the eggs and mix them in so they get combined with the veggies.

Sprinkle the kale crumbs over the top.

Heat your frying pan on a medium heat and let the frittata cook.

Flip over once crispy on the bottom, or pop the frying pan under a medium grill,
to cook the top.

Season with a little salt and pepper (for toddlers and adults only).

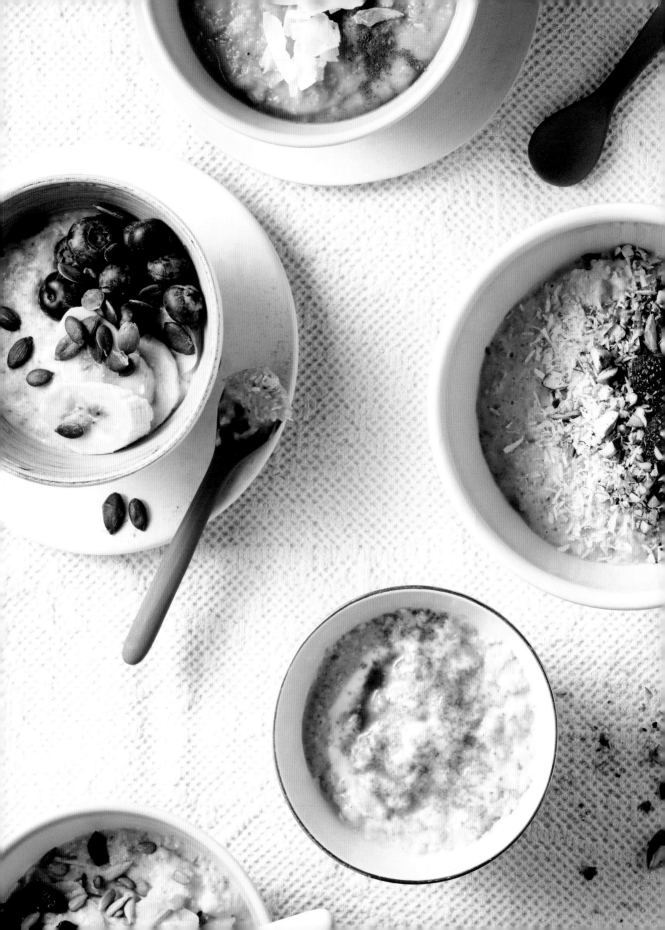

4 WAYS WITH PORRIDGE

Preparation time: 2 minutes
Chilling time: overnight (optional)
Cooking time: 3–4 minutes
Serves: 2

To buy:
any fresh or dried fruit,
   nuts or seeds for your
   flavour ingredients

Store-cupboard essentials:
100g porridge oats
125ml milk
125ml water
1 tablespoon honey (or maple
   syrup if serving to baby under
   1 year)

Mix the oats, milk, water and honey in a bowl and leave
in the fridge overnight, or cook straight away.

Pour the oat mixture into a pan and heat through for
3-4 minutes (cook for slightly longer if you didn't soak the
oats overnight).

Add extra milk to loosen the porridge to your desired
consistency.

Flavour your porridge with any of the combinations below.

Flavour ingredients:
♦ raspberry, pistachio and unsweetened desiccated coconut
♦ grated apple, cranberry and sunflower seeds
♦ banana, blueberry and pumpkin seeds
♦ pumpkin pie (coconut milk, pumpkin purée, cinnamon
♦ honey or maple syrup and cinnamon

MINI FRITTATA BITES

Preparation time: 10 minutes
Cooking time: 20–25 minutes
Makes: approx. 12

To buy:
½ tablespoon grated Cheddar
   cheese per muffin
an assortment of veggies and meats,
   e.g. grated courgettes, grated
   carrots, mushrooms, kale crumbs,
   spring onions, chopped tomatoes,
   cooked chicken, ham …

Store-cupboard essentials:
6 eggs
2 tablespoons milk
½ tablespoon grated Parmesan
   cheese per muffin

Preheat the oven to 200°C/gas 6.

Beat the eggs and milk and set aside.

Grease a mini muffin tray, then add the cheeses and the chopped
veg or meat in any combo you like.

Pour the egg mixture over the veggies.

Bake for 20-25 minutes, or until the eggs are fluffy and set.

Leave to cool on a cooling rack.

Tip: These can be frozen and reheated in
a microwave for the perfect speedy snack.

BUBBLE AND SQUEAK

Preparation time: 5 minutes
Cooking time: 10 minutes
Serves: 2

To buy:
2 handfuls any of roasted
  leftover vegetables
a handful of cooked meat

Store-cupboard essentials:
1 knob of butter
2 eggs
a handful of grated Parmesan cheese
salt and pepper, to taste

Turn your oven to a medium grill setting.

Melt the butter in a large frying pan on a medium heat.

Add the vegetables to the pan in an even layer, and top with
the cooked meat.

Crack the eggs over the vegetables and meat and sprinkle
with the cheese.

Cook for 5 minutes, then place under the grill for 2–4 minutes,
until the eggs are cooked to your liking and the cheese has melted.

Remove a portion for baby, then season with salt and pepper
(for toddlers and adults) before serving.

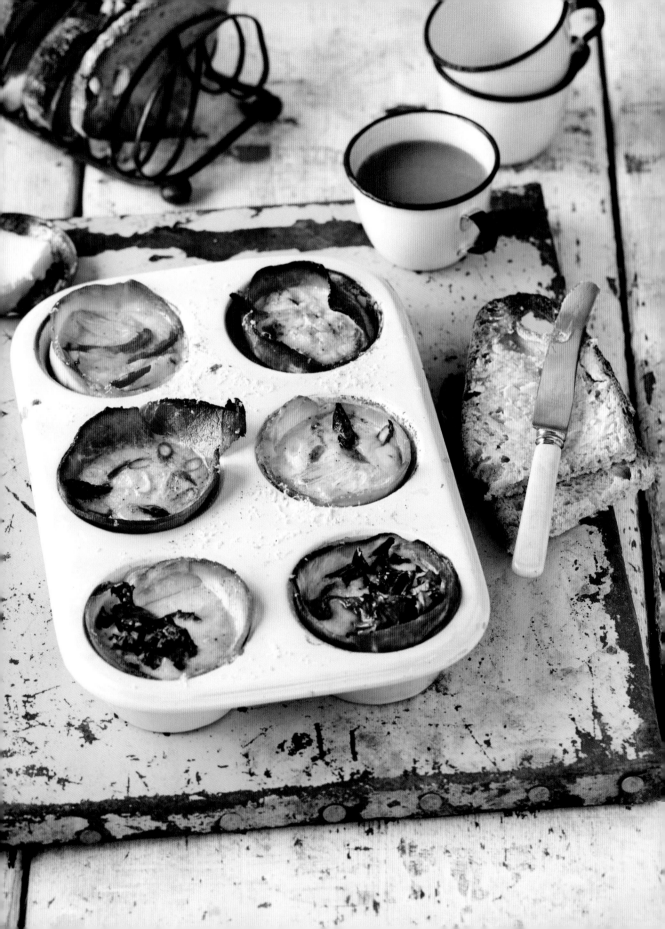

TURKEY AND HAM MUFFINS

Preparation time: 10 minutes
Cooking time: 20–25 minutes
Serves: 4–6

To buy:
6 slices of turkey or ham
any veggies you might have
   in the fridge, e.g. spinach,
   grated carrots, grated
   courgettes . . .

Store-cupboard essentials:
butter or olive oil, for greasing
6 eggs
6 tablespoons milk
50g grated Parmesan cheese, plus
   extra for sprinkling
salt and pepper, to taste

Preheat your oven to 200°C/gas 6.

Take a muffin tray and grease it with butter or olive oil.

Place a slice of turkey or ham in each muffin hole to form your 'muffin case'.

Beat the eggs, milk and Parmesan in a bowl.

Scoop out a portion for baby, then season the remainder with salt and pepper (for toddlers and adults).

Divide the egg mixture equally between the 6 cases. Sprinkle with a little Parmesan and any veggies.

Bake for 20-25 minutes, until the eggs are cooked through.

SWEET POTATO CRUSTLESS QUICHE

Preparation time: 15 minutes
Cooking time: 25–30 minutes
Serves: 6–8

To buy:
1 large sweet potato (approx.
   350-400g), washed and peeled
150g leftover cooked meat
100g feta or any hard cheese
300ml single cream

Store-cupboard essentials:
olive oil
salt and pepper, to taste
4 eggs
a handful of Kale Crumbs (see
   page 26) or fresh herbs

Preheat the oven to 180°C/gas 4 and grease a 20cm shallow pie dish with olive oil.

Slice the potato very thinly, either using a mandolin or by hand, and place
in a bowl.

Toss the sliced potato in a little olive oil and season with salt (omit if serving to baby) and pepper.

Layer the sweet potato across the bottom of a pie dish and around the edges to form a base.

Cut the meat and cheese into small cubes and layer on top of the sweet potato.

Beat the eggs and cream together, then add the kale crumbs.

Pour the mixture gently into the prepared pie dish.

Bake for 25-30 minutes, until set - don't overcook, as the eggs may scramble.

Leave to cool slightly before serving. Also delicious served cold.

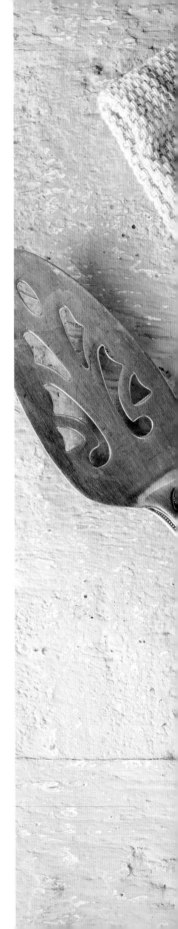

Tip: There are plenty of other fillings you can use, such as leftover cooked broccoli or fish.

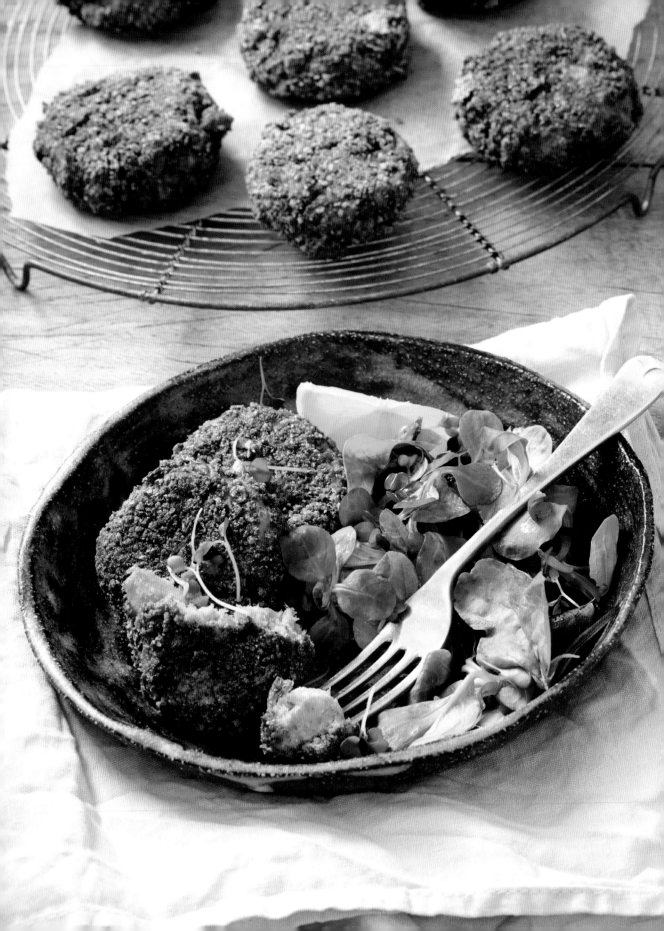

SALMON AND SWEET POTATO FISHCAKES

Preparation time: 15 minutes
Cooking time: 25–30 minutes
Makes: 12

To buy:
1 sweet potato, approx. 250g
250g salmon fillet
2 large handfuls of frozen peas
zest of 1 lemon

Store-cupboard essentials:
whole milk (enough to cover the fish,
   potato and peas)
salt and pepper, to taste
2 eggs
3 handfuls of breadcrumbs
olive oil

Preheat the oven to 190°C/gas 5 and line a baking tray with parchment paper.

Peel the sweet potato and cut into 1cm cubes.

Cut the salmon into cubes, making sure there are no bones.

Place the sweet potato, salmon and peas in a pan and cover with milk.

Heat on a medium heat and once the milk begins to boil, reduce to a simmer for 5–8 minutes, until the sweet potato is soft and the fish is cooked through.

Drain the milk (at this point you can remove a portion for baby, as it has no seasoning, and loosen with some of the poaching milk).

Mash the fish, sweet potato and peas and season with salt and pepper.

Stir in 1 egg quickly, so it doesn't scramble, and add the lemon zest.

Beat the remaining egg in a shallow dish, season with salt and set aside.

Place the breadcrumbs in a separate shallow dish.

Form the fish mash mixture into little patties, using your hands. Dip them first into the egg mixture and then into the crackers, and place on the lined baking tray.

Drizzle with a little olive oil.

Bake for 20 minutes, until golden brown, turning them over halfway through.

Pizza slices

Take a whole baked potato and cut it into slices about 1cm thick.

Place on a baking tray and top each slice with tomato passata or our Tomato Sauce with Hidden Vegetables (see page 231), mozzarella and toppings of your choice.

Place under the grill for a few minutes until the cheese has melted, then serve.

Jacket potato bombs

Preheat the oven to 180°C/gas 4.

Cut a cooked potato in half and scoop out the inside, leaving a shell.

Place some chopped ham and ricotta cheese in the empty skins, making sure you leave enough room for an egg. Then gently break an egg into each.

Place on a baking tray and cook in the oven for 15–20 minutes until the egg is cooked to your liking.

Sprinkle with herbs or seasoning of your choice.

4 WAYS WITH JACKET POTATOES

Sweet hasselbacks

Preheat the oven to 220°C/gas 7.

Cut a sweet potato almost all the way through, into thin horizontal slices.

Drizzle with olive oil.

Bake for 30–40 minutes.

Serve with a different filling:
- Ricotta, tomatoes and basil
- Avocado, cooked chicken and lemon
- Tuna and chopped red pepper mixed with Fool's Mayo (see page 91)
- Feta, sun-dried tomatoes and olive (not suitable for baby)
- Ham, goat's cheese and honey (not suitable for baby)

A twist from the normal

Try some of these alternative ideas to your regular baked potato:

- Chickpeas in tomato passata or our Tomato Sauce with Hidden Vegetables (see page 231) instead of baked beans.
- Fool's Mayo (see page 91).
- Kale Crumbs (see page 26) instead of herbs.
- Beetroot Blitz (see page 91) mixed with the mashed potato – bright and colourful.

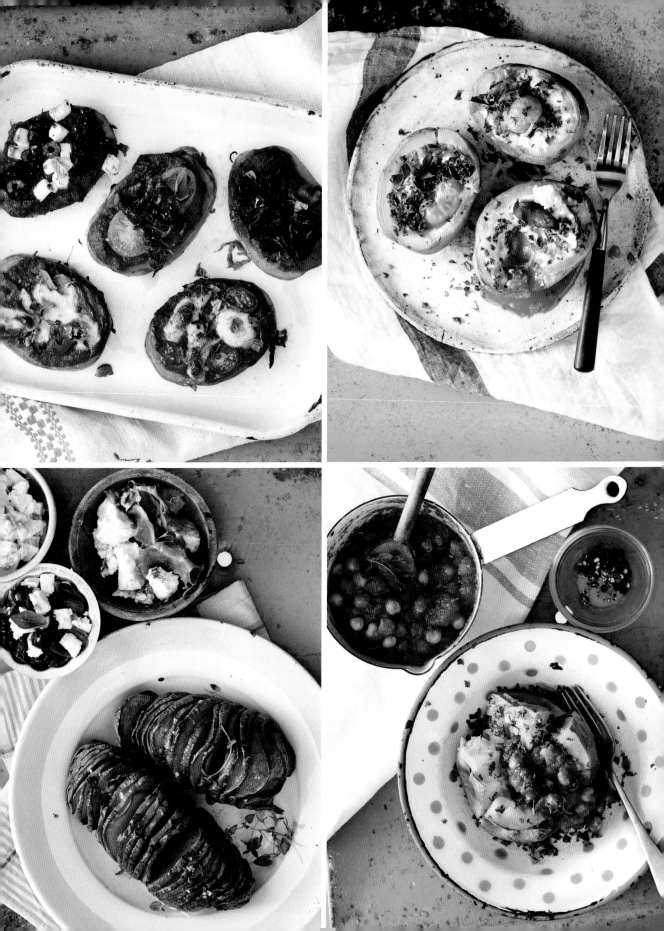

BROCCOLI BALLS

Preparation time: 15 minutes
Cooking time: 30–40 minutes
Makes: 12–16

To buy:
1 medium sweet potato (350g)
1 head of broccoli (350g)
a handful of cornflakes (40g)
1 teaspoon fresh or dried thyme

Store-cupboard essentials:
1 clove of garlic
a handful of pistachio nuts (40g)
3-4 handfuls of breadcrumbs
olive oil, for greasing
1 egg
4 heaped tablespoons grated Parmesan cheese (40g)
salt and pepper, to taste

Preheat the oven to 200°C/gas 6.

Peel and dice the sweet potato and cut the broccoli into florets.

Place in a steamer along with the peeled clove of garlic.

Steam the veg for 10-15 minutes, until soft, then leave to one side.

Blitz together the cornflakes and pistachio nuts using a blender and pot attachment and put aside into a small bowl.

Blitz together the breadcrumbs, broccoli, garlic, thyme, sweet potato, egg and Parmesan.

Remove a portion for baby then season the rest with salt and pepper.

Grease a baking tray with a little olive oil.

Roll into small balls and coat in the cornflake/pistachio mix, then place on the prepared tray and drizzle with a little olive oil.

Bake for 20-25 minutes, or until golden brown, turning after 15 minutes.

Serve hot or cold.

Tips: For a change, substitute the broccoli with 2 handfuls of frozen peas or spinach. Use an ice-cream scoop to measure out the balls on to the baking tray.

Stick toothpicks into the unseasoned balls to distinquish baby's from the others.

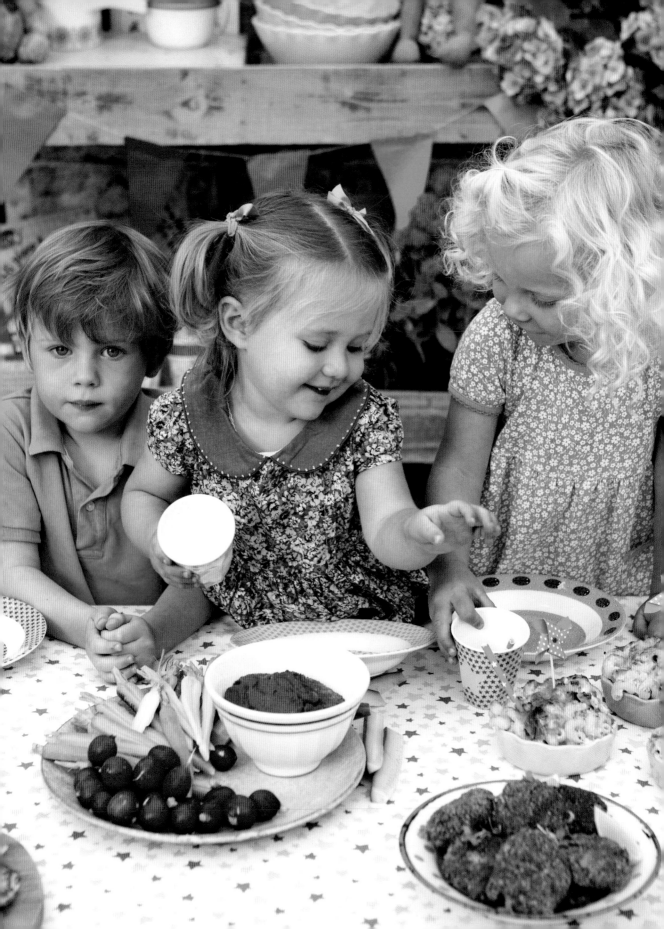

AUBERGINE BALLS

Preparation time: 15 minutes
Cooking time: 25 minutes
Makes: 12–16

To buy:
1 aubergine (about 250g)
a few leaves of fresh basil or
   ½ teaspoon dried basil

Store-cupboard essentials:
1 clove of garlic
1 egg
3-4 handfuls of breadcrumbs
4 heaped tablespoons grated
   Parmesan cheese (40g)
1 teaspoon dried oregano
salt and pepper, to taste
olive oil, for baking

Preheat the oven to 200°C/gas 6.

Wash and dice the aubergines, keeping the skin on, and place in a steamer along with the peeled clove of garlic.

Steam the aubergine for 15 minutes, until soft. Leave to cool slightly.

Blitz together the aubergine, garlic, egg, breadcrumbs, Parmesan, basil and oregano using a stick blender or pot attachment.

Set aside a portion for baby, then season with salt and pepper for toddlers and adults.

Grease a baking tray with a little olive oil.

Roll the aubergine mixture into small balls (using an ice-cream scoop makes this much easier) and place on the baking tray.

Drizzle them with a light coating of olive oil.

Bake for 20-25 minutes, or until golden brown, turning after 15 minutes.

Serve hot or cold.

Tip: You can add 2 tablespoons of Secret Sprinkles (see page 157) to add some texture.

RAINBOW RICOTTA GNOCCHI

Preparation time: 30 minutes
Cooking time: 2–3 minutes
Serves: 3–4

To buy:
500g ricotta
100g '00' flour, plus extra for dusting
  (you could also use plain flour)
polenta/semolina, for dusting

Store-cupboard essentials:
1 large egg
50g grated Parmesan cheese
salt, to taste (omit if serving
  to baby)

Line a bowl with several layers of kitchen paper and spoon the ricotta into the bowl. Let it drain for at least 30 minutes, or overnight in the fridge.

Mix the egg, Parmesan and a pinch of salt together, then mix in the ricotta.

Sift the flour over the ricotta mixture, adding any 'colour ingredient' (see below), and gently stir until all is incorporated. If you want more than one colour, don't forget to divide your ricotta mixture before adding your colour ingredient.

Dust the work surface with flour and roll a small amount of dough into sausage shapes – the smaller the better. Use extra flour to help roll into shape as the dough can be quite wet.

Cut the dough into small, even pieces, approximately 1cm long.

Sprinkle some polenta or semolina on to baking trays and place the gnocchi on them. Try not to overcrowd the trays so the gnocchi don't stick together. Continue until all the ricotta mix has been used up.

Cook the gnocchi in a large pot of salted boiling water until they float to the surface, about 2-3 minutes depending on the size of them.

Drain and serve with a sauce of your choice – we like either a melted butter and sage sauce or simply toss over some extra virgin olive oil and grated Parmesan.

Optional colour ingredients
(per 500g ricotta)

Pink = 1 teaspoon beetroot powder
Green = 1 tablespoon Kale Crumbs
  (see page 26)

Yellow = a large pinch of saffron powder
Black = 1 packet of squid ink
Orange = 1 tablespoon tomato purée

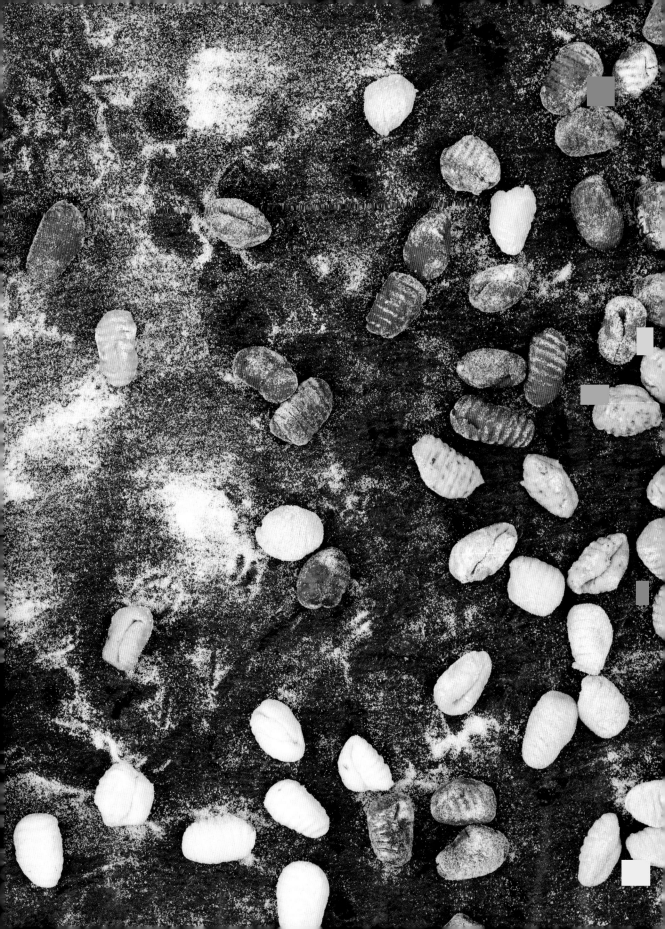

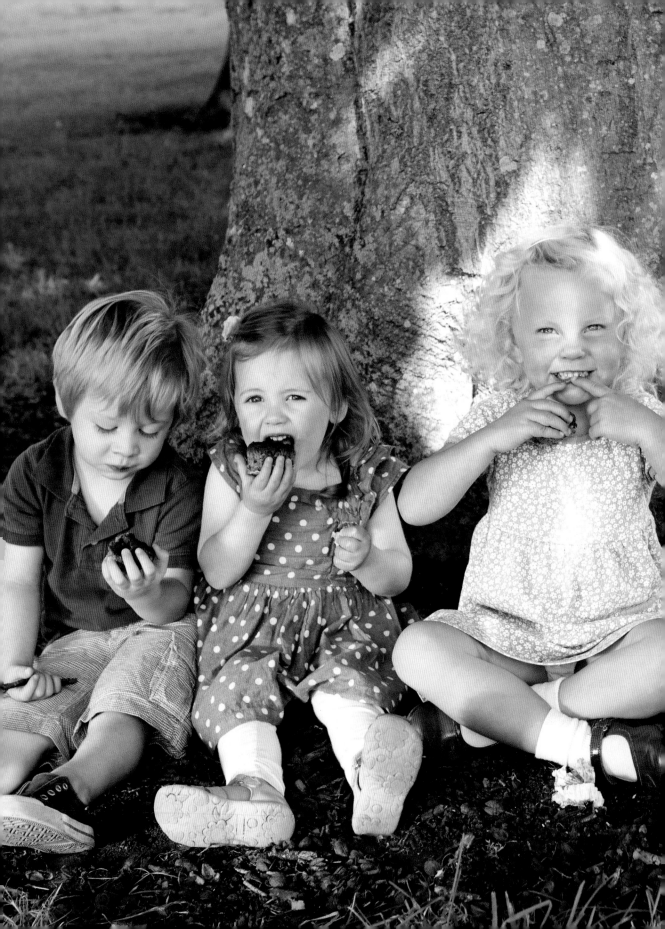

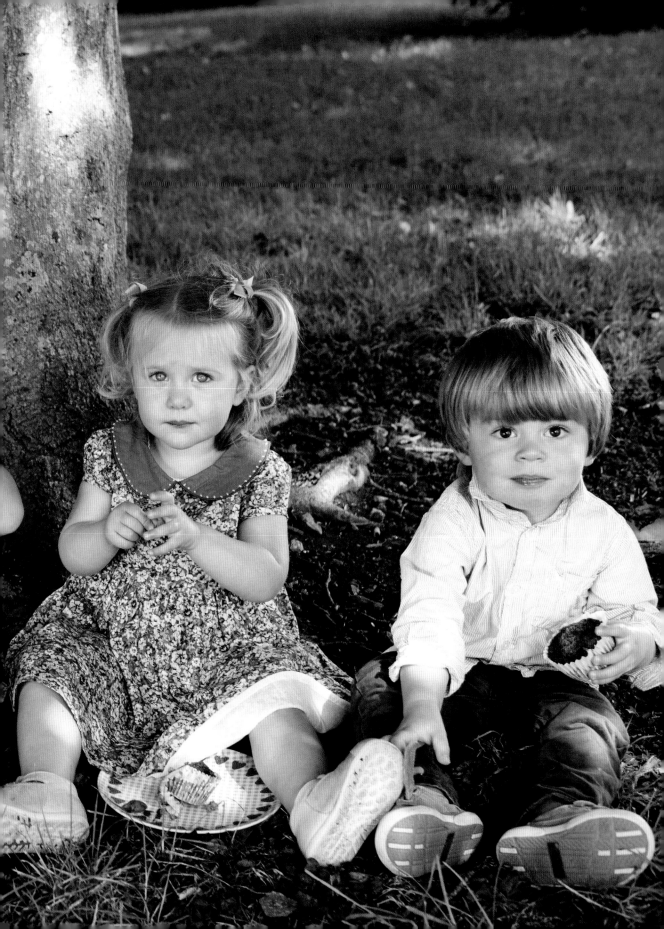

Leftover roasted veggies = veggie frittata:

Mash up leftover veggies and add to a frittata (see page 179).

Tip: Leftover veggies can also be added to a soup or stew.

Leftover bread = croutons:

Cut the bread into cubes, **drizzle** with olive oil and herbs of your liking and some salt flakes then **bake** in the oven at 200°C/gas 6 until crisp and golden brown (leave out the salt if feeding baby).

4 WAYS WITH LEFTOVERS

Leftover meat from roast = meatballs:

Mince or finely chop any leftover meat.

Add 1 egg, 1 tablespoon breadcrumbs, 1 tablespoon grated Parmesan and some herbs of your choice to every 4-5 tablespoons of leftover meat.

Season with salt (omit if serving to baby).

Mix it all together and roll into walnut-size meatballs.

Fry in a pan with a little olive oil until golden or bake in the oven at 200°C/gas 6 for 15-20 minutes, or until cooked through.

Leftover risotto = risotto fritters:

Add 1 egg, 1 tablespoon flour and a handful of grated cheese (we prefer Parmesan but Cheddar works too) to every 4-5 tablespoons of leftover risotto and mix well.

Heat a saucepan with a little butter and olive oil and dollop in spoonfuls of the risotto mixture to make little patties. Flatten with the back of a spoon, then flip once the bottoms have turned golden.

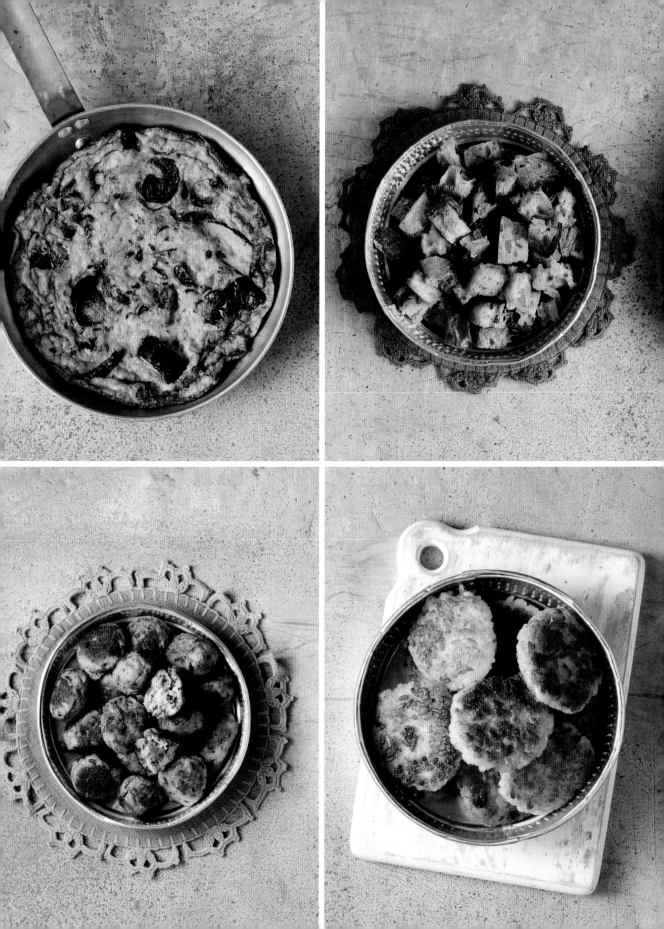

4 WAYS WITH PESTO

Tip: Any of these pestos can be stored in the fridge for several weeks – just make sure you cover the pesto with a layer of olive oil so that it stays fresh. They can also be frozen in ice-cube trays.

4 things to do with pesto

♦ Scrambled in eggs

♦ Drizzled over fish

♦ Sautéed with veg

♦ Spread on toast with ham and cheese

Pea, walnut and mint pesto

To buy:
2 handfuls of peas (fresh or frozen)
a handful of fresh mint
juice of 1 lemon

Store-cupboard essentials:
2 handfuls of walnuts
1 clove of garlic
8 tablespoons extra virgin olive oil
2 handfuls of grated Parmesan
cheese (30g)
salt and pepper, to taste

Courgette, lemon and parsley pesto

To buy:
½ a grated courgette
a handful of fresh parsley
juice of ½ a lemon

Store-cupboard essentials:
50g cashews
1 clove of garlic
8 tablespoons extra virgin olive oil
2 handfuls of grated Parmesan
cheese (30g)
salt and pepper, to taste

Broccoli pesto

To buy:
½ a head of broccoli, cut into
small pieces
1 ripe avocado
juice of 1 lemon
a handful of fresh basil
1 tablespoon Kale Crumbs (see
page 26) (optional)

Store-cupboard essentials:
a handful of pine nuts, cashews
or chickpeas (20g)
1 clove of garlic
8 tablespoons extra virgin olive oil
2 handfuls of grated Parmesan
cheese (30g)
salt and pepper, to taste

Classic basil pesto

To buy:
2 handfuls of fresh basil

Store-cupboard essentials:
50g cashews
1 clove of garlic
8 tablespoons extra virgin olive oil
2 handfuls of grated Parmesan
cheese (30g)
salt and pepper, to taste

For each recipe:

Preparation time: 5-10 minutes
Serves: 6-8

Blitz all the ingredients together until smooth using a stick blender or pot attachment. Remove a portion for baby before seasoning for toddlers and adults.

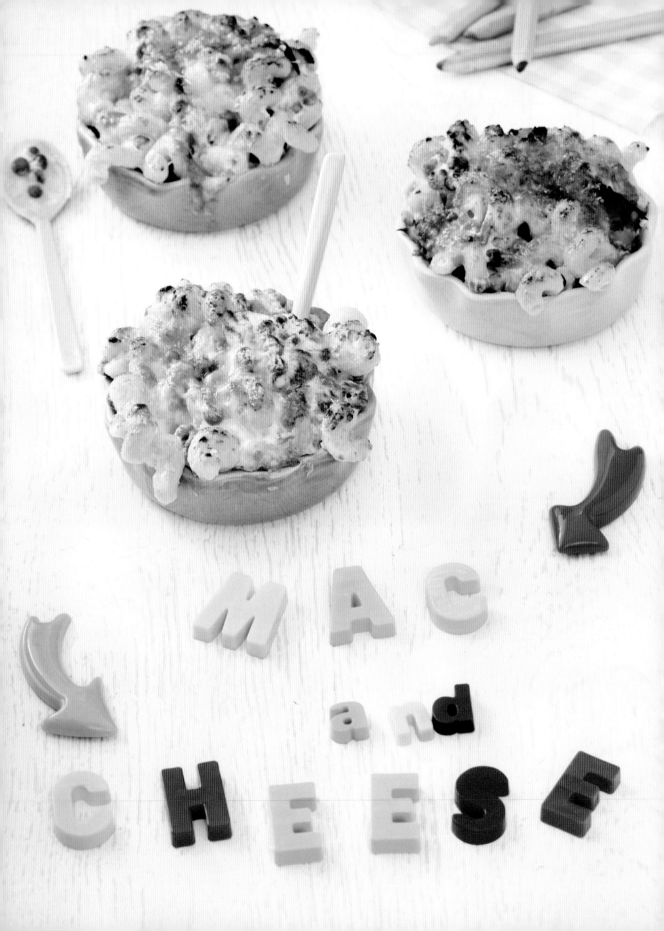

BAKED MAC AND CHEESE

Preparation time: 15 minutes
Cooking time: 10–15 minutes (depending on what pasta you use)
Serves: 4

To buy:
1 portion of Cheat's White Sauce (see page 90), using 250g ricotta and 70ml milk
salt, pepper and nutmeg, to taste
4 handfuls of peas
4 slices of ham

Store-cupboard essentials:
200g pasta
100g cheese of your choice (we like to use a mix of grated Cheddar, mozzarella and Parmesan)
a splash of milk

Cook the pasta in salted water until al dente.

Grate the cheese.

Drain the pasta and place in an ovenproof dish.

Stir in the Cheat's White Sauce, half the grated cheese and the peas.

Tear the ham into the pasta.

Remove a portion for baby, then season with salt, pepper and nutmeg and stir again.

Sprinkle the remaining cheese on top.

Pour a dash of milk into each corner of the dish to make sure it doesn't dry out in the oven.

Place under the grill for 5-10 minutes, until the cheese has melted and turned golden brown.

This is quite a rich recipe so perhaps keep it for a special treat.

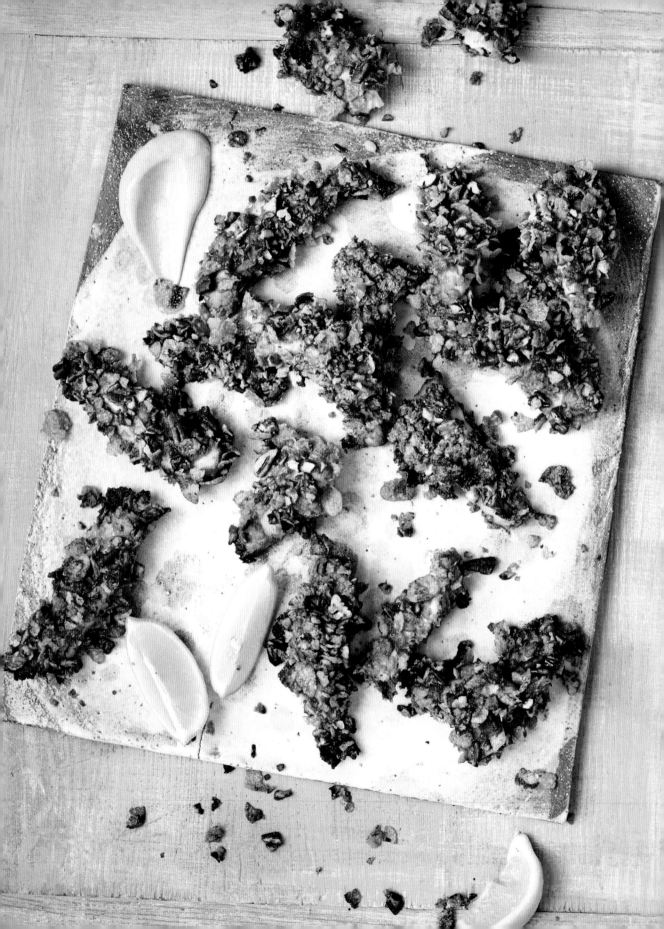

HEALTHY CRISPY CHICKEN TENDERS

Preparation time: 10 minutes
Cooking time: 20–25 minutes
Serves: 2–4

To buy:
2 boneless, skinless chicken breasts
4 tablespoons Greek yoghurt
1 tablespoon Dijon mustard (optional)
4 handfuls of cereal of your choice,
   free from added salt and sugar
   (e.g. cornflakes) (40g)

Store-cupboard essentials:
2 tablespoons honey (avoid if
   serving to baby under 1 year)
2 handfuls of chopped almonds or
   pecans (40g)
a drizzle of extra virgin olive oil
salt, to taste

Preheat the oven to 180°C/gas 4.

Line a baking tray with parchment paper or a non-stick mat and set aside.

Cut the chicken breasts into lengthways strips and pat dry with a paper towel, then set aside.

Stir together the Greek yoghurt, honey and Dijon mustard (if using) in a large bowl.

Place the chicken in the bowl and toss to coat each piece with yoghurt.

Crush the cereal and stir with the nuts in a shallow dish.

Dip each piece of yoghurt-coated chicken into the crumb mixture and coat evenly, then place on a baking tray.

Drizzle the chicken with olive oil and bake for 20-25 minutes, or until the chicken is thoroughly cooked, turning the pieces over after 10-15 minutes.

Serve with a squeeze of lemon and crushed salt flakes on top (omit the salt for baby).

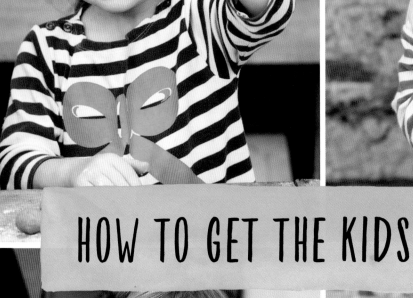
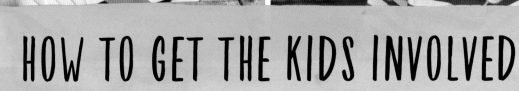

HOW TO GET THE KIDS INVOLVED

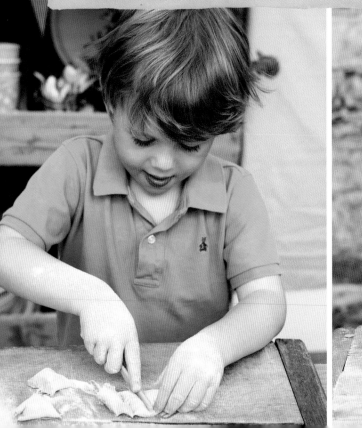
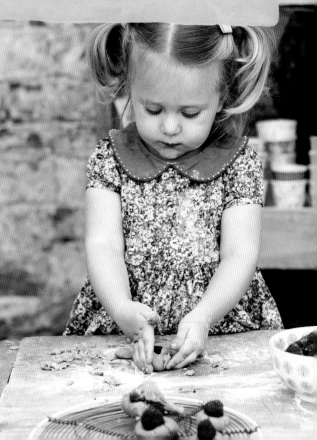

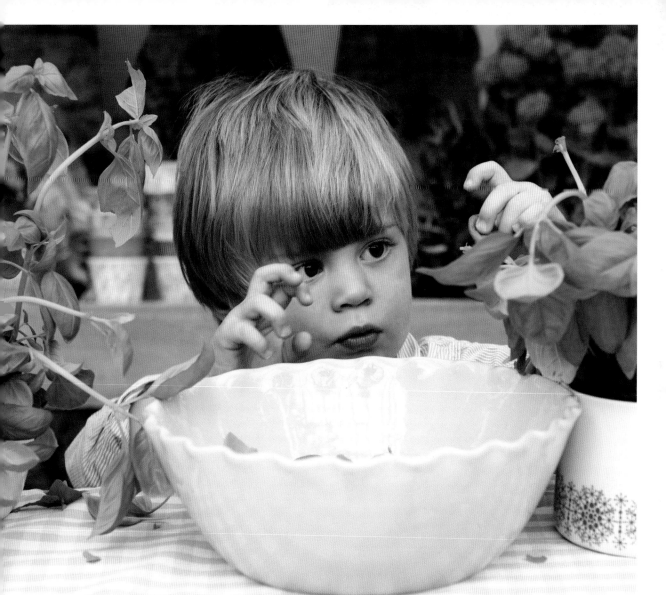

Gnocchi (see page 196):
Get your kids to help you roll out and cut the gnocchi.

Pesto (see page 202):
Get your kids to help you pick the basil leaves while you prepare dinner.

Beetroot Hummus (see page 118):
Get your kids to help squash the chickpeas between their fingers to take the skins off, which makes for a smoother hummus.

Buckwheat Jammy Dodgers and Ginger Nuts (see pages 143 and 152):
Get your kids to help you roll the dough and push their fingers into middle of the biscuits for the raspberries and almonds.

Broccoli and Aubergine Balls (see pages 192 and 195):
Get your kids to help you roll out the veggie balls.

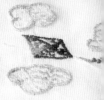

Tip: Best when filled with sauce to the top of the mug (otherwise the pastry sinks. Cut out 3 discs for the top of each mug for a really high puff.

FISH PIES IN A MUG

Preparation time: 10 minutes
Cooking time: 20–30 minutes
Serves: 4

To buy:

600–700g fish (salmon, white fillet
  or smoked haddock)
300ml crème fraîche
zest and juice of 1 lemon
fresh parsley (you can also use
  dill or thyme)
1 packet of pre-rolled puff pastry,
  approx. 320g

Store-cupboard essentials:

salt and pepper, to taste

Preheat the oven to 180°C/gas 4.

Cut the fish into approx. 3cm chunks.

Mix the fish with the crème fraîche in a medium bowl.

Add the zest and juice of the lemon to the fish.

Season with the herbs, remove a portion for baby, then add salt and pepper (for toddlers and adults) and set aside.

Use the top of a mug to cut out discs of puff pastry and set aside.

Pour the fish mixture evenly into 4 ovenproof mugs.

Place a pastry disc on top of each mug.

Bake in the oven for 20-30 minutes, or until the fish is cooked through and the pastry is golden.

Tip: All the soups in this section are suitable for freezing (before adding crème fraîche or yoghurt).

LEEK, POTATO AND PARSNIP SOUP

Preparation time: 5 minutes
Cooking time: 20 minutes
Serves: 6–8

To buy:
2 parsnips
2 sweet or white potatoes
2 leeks
500ml vegetable or chicken stock
fresh herbs to season, such as parsley,
   or Kale Crumbs (see page 26)

Store-cupboard essentials:
1 onion
salt and pepper, to taste

Peel and roughly chop all the washed vegetables.

Place all the vegetables in a large saucepan, pour over the stock and bring to the boil.

Simmer for 20 minutes.

Remove from the heat and leave to cool slightly.

Blitz with a stick blender until smooth, or leave some chunks if preferred.

Remove a portion for baby, then season to taste with salt (for toddlers and adults), pepper and some fresh herbs or kale crumbs, if desired.

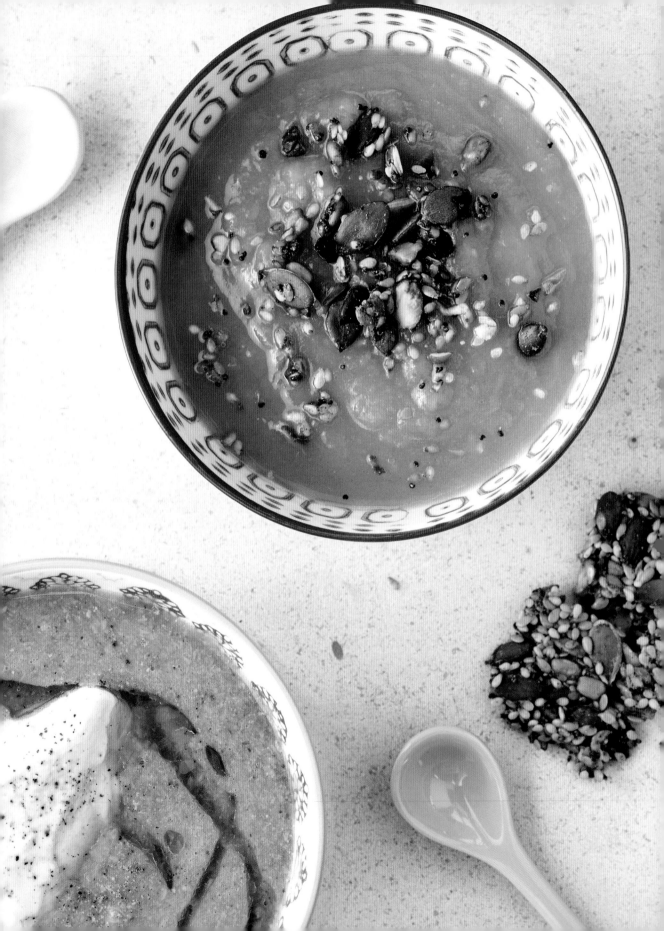

SIMPLE BUTTERNUT SQUASH SOUP

Preparation time: 5 minutes
Cooking time: 15–20 minutes
Serves: 6–8

Store-cupboard essentials:
1 medium onion, peeled
1 clove of garlic (optional)
salt and pepper, to taste

To buy:
1 medium butternut squash (approx. 1kg)
500ml vegetable or chicken stock

Tip: Try using some fresh grated ginger or turmeric to season.

Deseed the squash.

Cut the squash and onion into large chunks.

Place these in a large pan with the garlic, pour over the stock and bring to the boil.

Simmer for 20 minutes.

Remove from the heat and leave to cool slightly.

Blitz with a stick blender until smooth.

Remove a portion for baby, then season to taste, with salt (for toddlers and adults) and pepper.

BROCCOLI, PEA AND APPLE SOUP

Preparation time: 5 minutes
Cooking time: 20 minutes
Serves: 6–8

Store-cupboard essentials:
salt and pepper, to taste

To buy:
3 large eating apples
500g broccoli, broken into florets
500g frozen peas
500ml vegetable or chicken stock
fresh herbs, to season, such as parsley

Peel, core and roughly chop the apples.

Place all the vegetables and apples in a large saucepan, pour over the stock and bring to the boil.

Simmer for 20 minutes.

Remove from the heat and leave to cool slightly.

Blitz with a stick blender until smooth.

Remove a portion for baby, then season to taste, with salt (for toddlers and adults) and pepper and some fresh herbs, if desired.

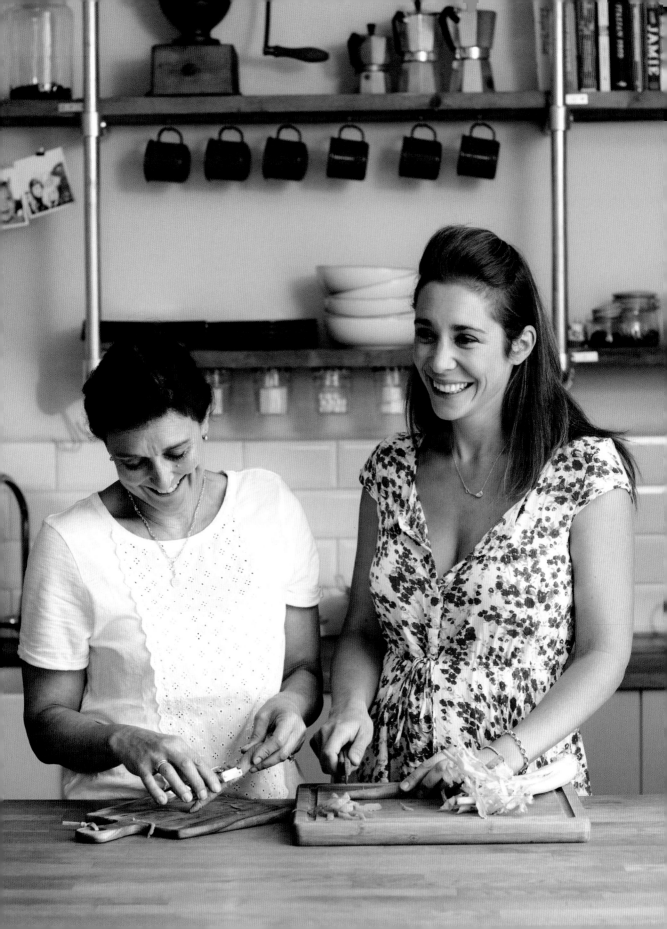

BEEF BOLOGNESE WITH HIDDEN VEGETABLES

Preparation time: 15 minutes
Cooking time: 1 hour
Serves: 6

To buy:
1 carrot
1 stick of celery
1 large uncooked beetroot, washed
500g minced beef

Store-cupboard essentials:
1 onion, cut in half
olive oil
1 clove of garlic
1 x 400g tin of chopped tomatoes
500ml boiling water
salt and pepper, to taste

Preheat your oven to 180°C/gas 4.

Place the carrot, celery, onion and beetroot on a baking tray and drizzle with olive oil.

Cook in the oven for approximately 45 minutes to 1 hour, until all the vegetables are roasted.

Heat a little olive oil in a large saucepan and, once hot, add the whole clove of garlic for a couple of minutes.

Add the mince, and once the meat is all brown, add the tinned tomatoes and the water and bring to the boil.

Simmer on a gentle heat for approximately 1 hour (around the time the vegetables are done).

Place the vegetables, once cooked, in a bowl and blitz them with a stick blender.

Add them to the saucepan with the minced meat.

Remove the whole clove of garlic.

Remove a portion for the baby, then season for the rest of the family with salt and pepper.

SOUP BOMB - POACH AN
EGG IN A BOWL OF SOUP

TURKEY AND HAM
MUFFINS (SEE PAGE 185)

4 WAYS WITH EGGS

BUBBLE AND SQUEAK
(SEE PAGE 183)

JACKET POTATO BOMB
(SEE PAGE 190)

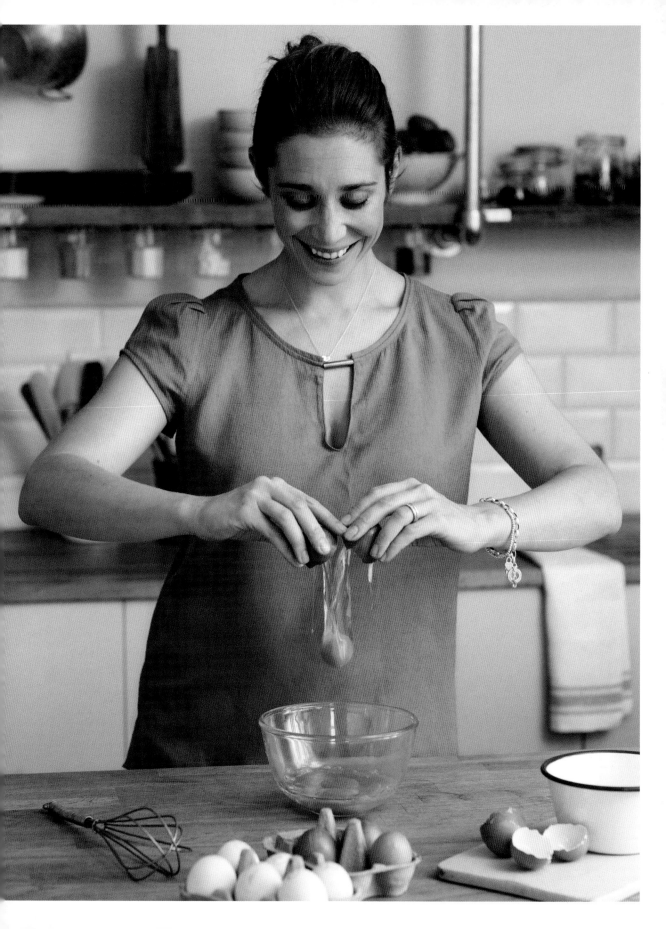

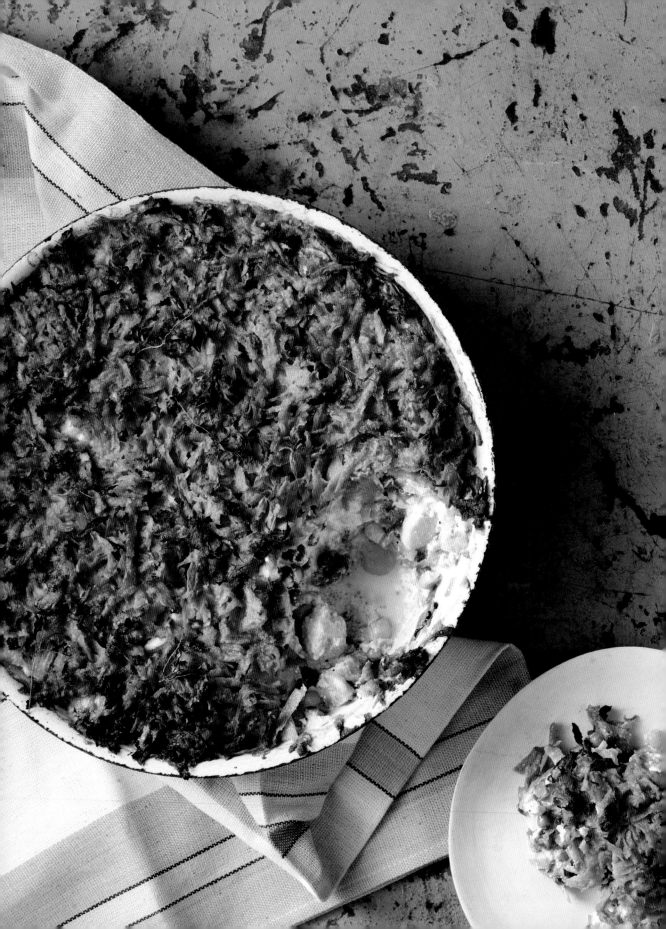

CHICKEN POT PIE

Preparation time: 15 minutes
Cooking time: 40–50 minutes
Serves: 6

To buy:
2 medium sweet potatoes
450g chicken breast (or cold
    leftover chicken), chopped into
    1cm cubes
1 leek, trimmed, washed and
    finely chopped
2 x 250g tubs of ricotta
grated nutmeg (optional)
8 handfuls of frozen peas (165g)
165g drained tinned sweetcorn

Store-cupboard essentials:
3 tablespoons olive oil, plus extra
    for drizzling
herbs of your choice (e.g. thyme sprigs,
    parsley, etc.)
salt and pepper, to taste
1 tablespoon butter
200ml milk

Preheat your oven to 180°C/gas 4.

Wash the sweet potatoes and grate with skins on into a bowl.

Toss with 2 tablespoons of olive oil and the herbs and put to one side.

Heat 1 tablespoon of olive oil and the butter in a frying pan.

Add the chicken cubes and leeks and cook for 10 minutes, then remove from the heat.

Mix together the ricotta and milk and place the ricotta mix, cooked chicken and leek, frozen peas and sweetcorn in a large ovenproof dish. Stir gently to combine.

Top with the grated sweet potato and drizzle with olive oil.

Bake for 30-40 minutes, until bubbling and crispy on top.

Remove a portion for baby, then season the rest with salt, pepper and nutmeg, if using.

Tips: A great recipe for using up leftover chicken from Sunday lunch.
Try also using different meats, like turkey or pork.

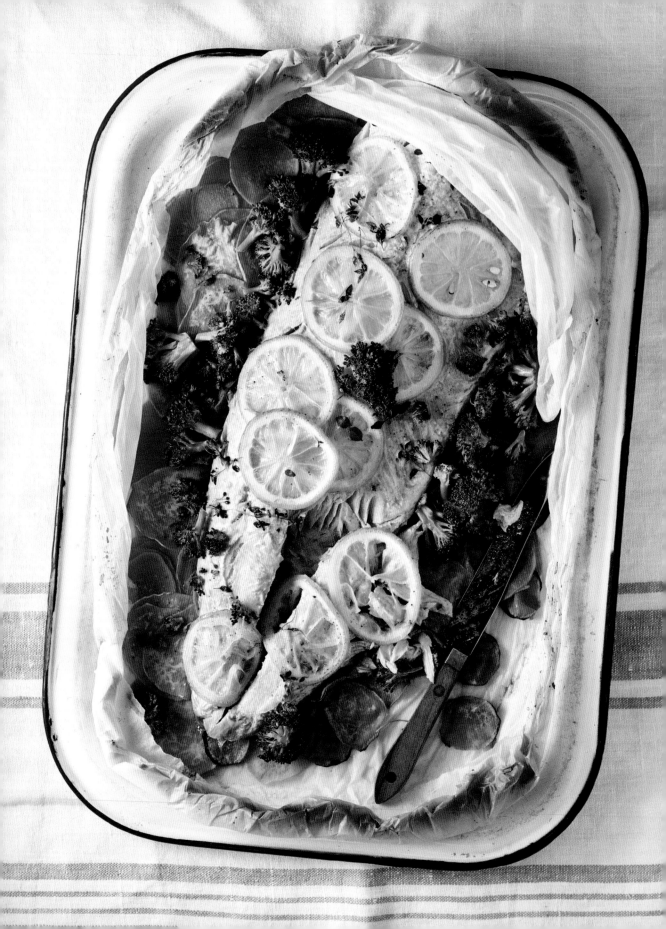

SALMON AND SWEET POTATO PARCEL

Preparation time: 15 minutes
Cooking time: 25 minutes
Serves: 4

To buy:
1 whole salmon fillet (approx. 600–700g)
2 sweet potatoes
1 lemon
2–3 sprigs of fresh thyme (or other herbs
   of choice)
1 head of broccoli

Store-cupboard essentials:
1–2 tablespoons extra virgin olive oil
salt and pepper, to taste

Preheat the oven to 200°C/gas 6.

Cut two large pieces of baking parchment, big enough to fit the salmon and have a border of at least 10cm around the fish. Place one sheet on a baking tray and set the other aside.

Wash and dry the sweet potatoes, then, using a mandolin or sharp knife, cut them into very thin circular slices.

Cut the lemon into thin slices and set aside.

Arrange the sweet potato slices in the middle of the parchment paper to create a base for the fish to sit on. Set the fish on top of the potatoes.

Place the lemon slices on top of the fish, and scatter the thyme and broccoli florets over and around it.

Drizzle all over with extra virgin olive oil and season with salt (for toddlers and adults only) and pepper.

Top the fish with the second piece of parchment and, starting at one corner, twist the edges of both sheets all the way round to seal the parcel. Make sure there aren't any gaps for the steam to escape, otherwise the sweet potatoes won't cook properly.

Cook in the oven for 25 minutes – do not open the parcel before the time is up.

CHEAT'S RISOTTO

Preparation time: 10 minutes
Cooking time: 20 minutes
Serves: 2–3

To buy:
1 courgette
1 carrot
800ml chicken stock (see page 227)
6 slices of ham
3 tablespoons ricotta

Store-cupboard essentials:
250g Arborio rice
30g grated Parmesan cheese, plus extra to serve
salt and pepper, to taste

Grate the courgette and carrot, using the wide teeth on a cheese grater.

Add the rice, stock, grated courgette and carrot to a large pan and turn on the heat (there's no need to wait for the stock to boil before adding the ingredients).

Boil for approximately 15-20 minutes until the rice is cooked. Check by tasting a few grains; it should be soft but with a slight bite.

Chop the ham into small pieces.

Drain the rice, courgette and carrot and return to the hot pan.

Stir in the ricotta, Parmesan and ham.

Mix well to combine. Remove a portion for baby, then season, to taste, with salt (for toddlers and adults) and pepper.

Serve immediately, topped with extra grated Parmesan.

4-BEAN FEAST

Preparation time: 15 minutes
Cooking time: 30 minutes
Serves: 6

To buy:
1 carrot
2 sweet potatoes
100g green beans
400ml vegetable stock

Store-cupboard essentials:
1 onion
2 tablespoons olive oil
1 x 400g tin of red kidney beans
1 x 400g tin of cannellini beans
1 x 400g tin of borlotti beans
1 x 400g tin of chopped tomatoes
1 tablespoon each of chopped
  basil and oregano

Preheat the oven to 200°C/gas 6.

Chop the vegetables into chunks.

Heat the oil in a large ovenproof pan and fry the fresh veg for
a few minutes.

Drain and rinse all the tinned beans and add to the pot.

Add the tomatoes, herbs and vegetable stock and stir to combine.

Cover with a lid and place in the oven.

Cook for 30 minutes.

Remove a portion for baby, then season with salt and pepper for toddlers
and adults

Tip: Great served over a jacket potato or
blitzed to make a hearty soup.

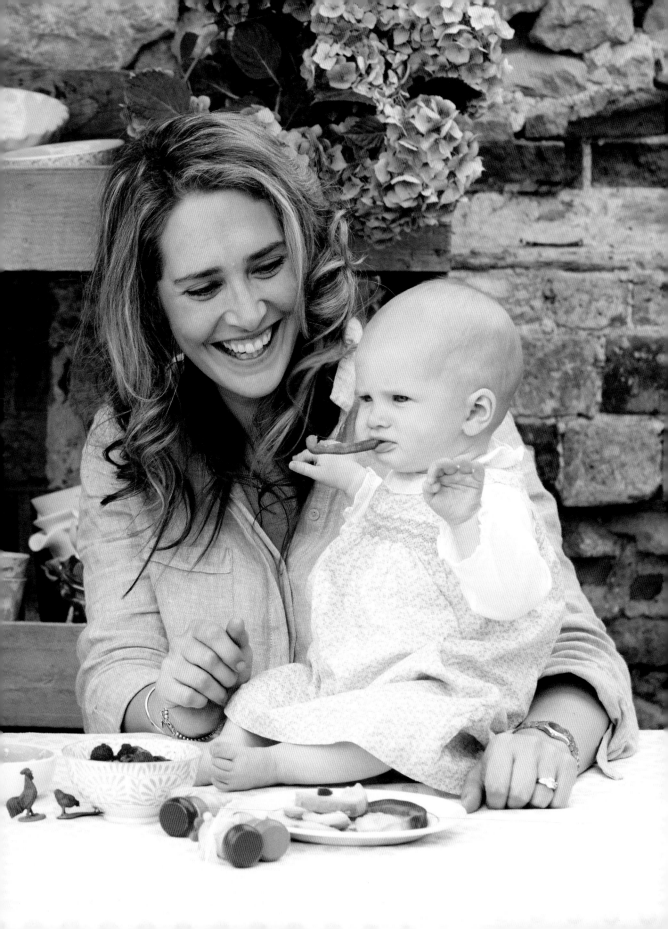

BONE BROTH AND CHICKEN BALLS

Preparation time: 15 minutes
Cooking time: 3 hours
Serves: 6–8

To buy:
1 carrot
1 stick of celery
1kg chicken thighs (with bones)

Store-cupboard essentials:
1 onion, peeled
200g breadcrumbs
6-8 tablespoons grated Parmesan cheese
1 egg
1 tablespoon chopped herbs (oregano,
    thyme or parsley)
salt and pepper, to taste
plain flour, for coating
olive oil

Place all the veg and chicken in a large pan of water over a high heat, and once it's boiling, lower to a simmer. Make sure the water is covering the chicken and veg. There's no need to chop the veg beforehand.

Simmer for a minimum of 2-3 hours.

Strain through a fine mesh sieve, keeping the meat, carrot, celery and onion to one side.

Pour into a container and store in the fridge or freeze for future use.

Strip all the meat from the chicken bones and add to the breadcrumbs.

Add the grated Parmesan, egg, herbs and the cooked carrot, onion and celery.

Blitz all together, remove a portion for baby, then season with salt (for toddlers and adults) and pepper.

Roll into small balls the size of walnuts.

Fry in a large pan or bake on a tray with a little olive oil till golden brown, and serve.

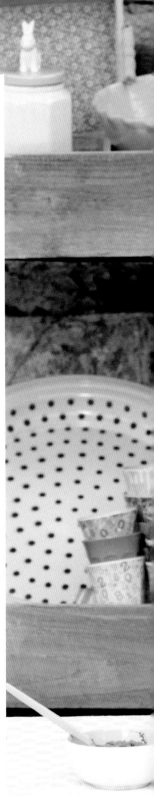

MAKE-AHEAD MEALS

The following are meals that we always make a double batch of so that we can put the extras in the freezer and have a ready-made meal to just heat up in the oven or microwave at any time.

SALMON AND SWEET POTATO FISHCAKES (SEE PAGE 189)

. . . .

RAINBOW RICOTTA GNOCCHI (SEE PAGE 196)

. . . .

CHICKEN POT PIE (SEE PAGE 221)

. . . .

RED PEPPER AND SUPER-BEAN BOLOGNESE (SEE PAGE 235)

. . . .

BONE BROTH (SEE PAGE 227)

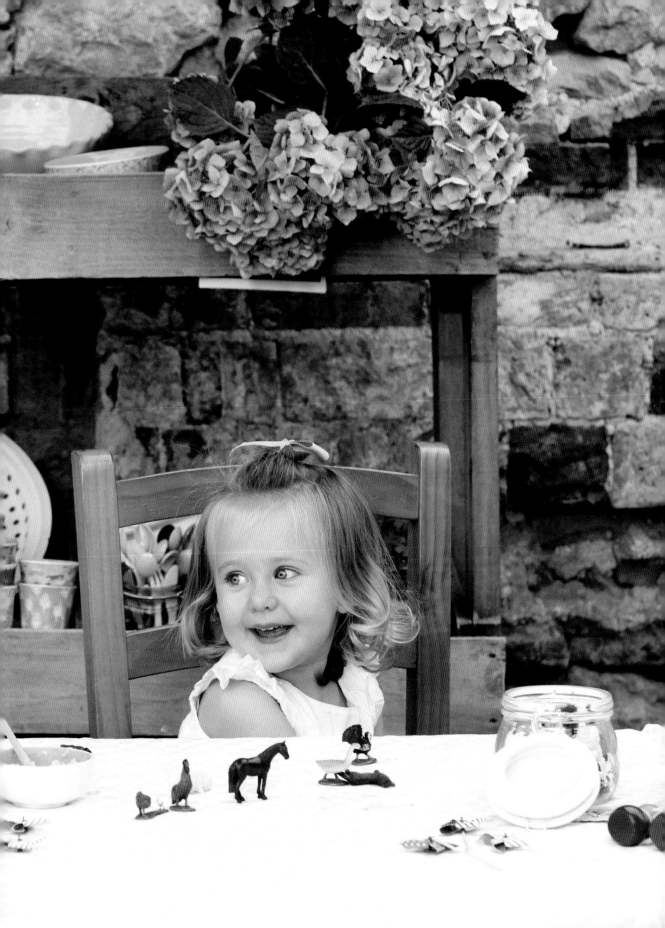

Tip: We have left fresh herbs out of this recipe in case you have a picky eater – however, a handful of parsley, basil or Kale Crumbs (see page 26) is a great addition.

TOMATO SAUCE WITH HIDDEN VEGETABLES

Preparation time: 10 minutes
Cooking time: 40 minutes
Serves: 6

To buy:
1 carrot
1 stick of celery
1 courgette
2 tablespoons tomato purée

Store-cupboard essentials:
1 onion
1 clove of garlic
2 x 400g tins of chopped tomatoes
500ml water
2 tablespoons extra virgin olive oil
salt and pepper, to taste

Wash and roughly chop the vegetables and place in a medium pan (no need to peel them).

Add the tinned tomatoes, water, olive oil and tomato purée.

Bring to the boil with the lid on for 10 minutes, then reduce to a simmer for 30–40 minutes with the lid off.

Remove from the heat and cool slightly.

Blitz with a stick blender until smooth and no pieces of vegetables are left.

Remove a portion for baby, then season with salt and pepper to taste (for toddlers and adults).

Serve over pasta, on a jacket potato, or add to soups and stews.

4 other uses for tomato sauce with hidden veg
♦ Serve over pasta as a sauce.
♦ Use as a pizza sauce on your dough.
♦ Add a cup to your soup for an extra vegetable boost.
♦ Use like a salsa dip – just add seasoning for toddlers and adults.

SALMON AND BROCCOLI PASTA

Preparation time: 5 minutes
Cooking time: 10 minutes
Serves: 6

To buy:
2 small heads of broccoli (approx. 150g)
250g cream cheese
zest and juice of 1 large lemon
300-400g cooked salmon, skinned
   and boned

Store-cupboard essentials:
salt and pepper, to taste
350g farfalle or other pasta

Bring a large pot of salted water to the boil over a high heat.

Cook the pasta in the boiling water according to the packet instructions.

Cut the broccoli into florets and add to the pasta 2 minutes before the end of the cooking time.

Drain the pasta and broccoli and put to one side, reserving a cup of the pasta water.

Place the cream cheese and lemon zest and juice in the same large pan and gently heat through.

Add the pasta, broccoli and flaked cooked salmon and coat with the cream sauce. If necessary, add some of the reserved pasta water to make a looser sauce.

Remove a portion for baby, then season with salt (for toddlers and adults) and pepper.

Tip: If your children don't like seeing the broccoli, add it to the pasta water 5 minutes before the pasta is cooked so that when you stir the sauce in, the broccoli disintegrates and is less visible.

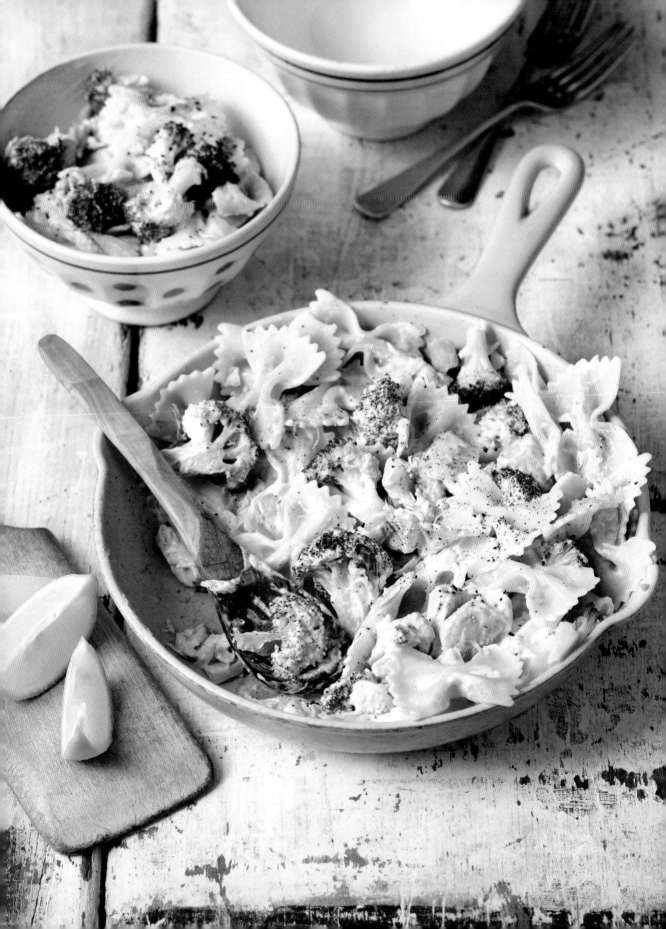

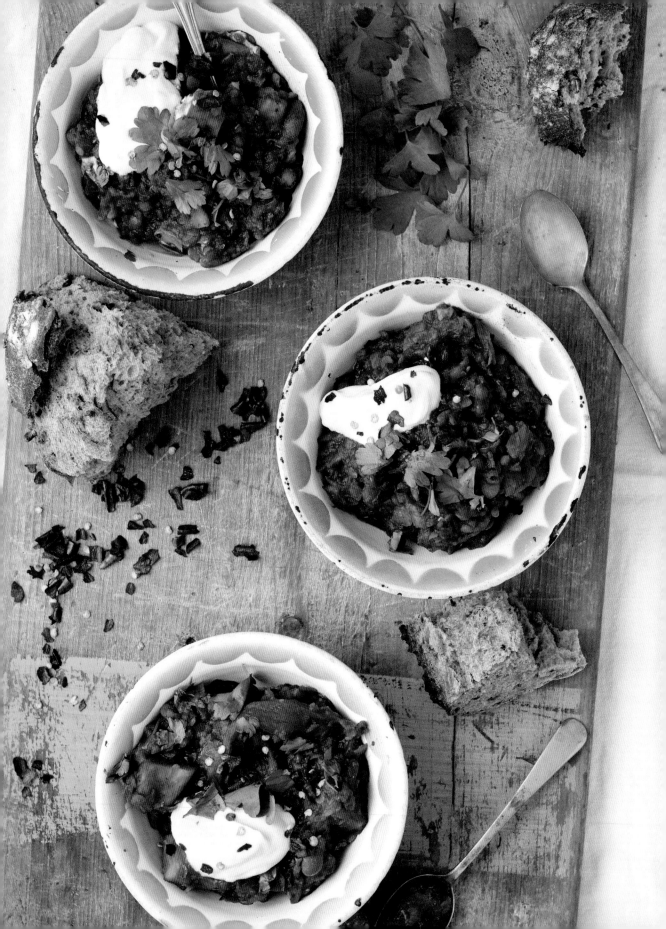

RED PEPPER AND SUPER-BEAN BOLOGNESE

Preparation time: 15 minutes
Cooking time: 1 hour
Serves: 8–10

To buy:
2 red peppers
2 sweet potatoes
1 litre vegetable stock
2 tablespoons sweet paprika
2 tablespoons tomato purée
2 tablespoons dried thyme

To serve: Greek yoghurt (optional)
fresh parsley (optional)
2 teaspoons chilli flakes (optional
  for adults)

Store-cupboard essentials:
2 medium onions
2 cloves of garlic
2 tablespoons olive oil
400g dried red lentils
2 x 400g tins of chopped tomatoes
2 x 400g tins of borlotti beans
  (or any other tinned bean)
2 tablespoons dried oregano
salt and pepper, to taste

Dice the onions, peppers and sweet potatoes and finely chop the garlic.

Place in a large heavy-based pan with the olive oil.

Cook for a few minutes, then add all the remaining ingredients except the yoghurt, parsley, chilli flakes and salt and pepper.

Stir well to combine, bring it all to the boil, then reduce to a low heat .

Cover with a lid and cook for 1 hour, stirring every 15 minutes to prevent it sticking.

Remove a portion for baby, then season with salt and pepper for toddlers and adults.

Serve with a dollop of Greek yoghurt, some freshly chopped parsley, and chilli flakes if serving to adults.

Tip: This recipe makes a large amount, but it freezes really well.

CHEESY CARROT CRACKERS

Preparation time: 10 minutes
Cooking time: 15–20 minutes
Serves: 6–8

To buy:
2 carrots

Store-cupboard essentials:
150g tasty hard cheese, e.g. Parmesan or Cheddar
120g plain flour (or alternative flour of your choice)
120g Secret Sprinkles (see page 157), or any seeds
   of your choice such as sunflower or flax
2 tablespoons olive oil
1 tablespoon dried oregano
salt and pepper, to taste

Preheat the oven to 180°C/gas 4.

Grate the carrots and cheese.

Blend all the ingredients until they resemble coarse breadcrumbs, seasoning with salt and pepper if making for toddlers and adults only. You may need to do this batches depending on the size of your pot attachment.

Pulse in 1-2 tablespoons of water, a tablespoon at a time, until it becomes a firm dough.

Roll the mixture out really thinly on a silicone mat or sheet of parchment paper and then place on to a baking tray.

Score the dough with a knife into equal portions or the shapes you want.

Bake for 15-20 minutes, until the crackers are hard and slightly brown.

Remove from the oven and allow to cool completely on the tray before eating.

ORANGE AND LEMON SEMOLINA DELIGHT

Preparation time: 5 minutes
Cooking time: 5 minutes
Makes: 4–6 mini portions

To buy:
100g semolina
200ml orange juice
zest and juice of 1 lemon,
    plus extra zest to garnish

Store-cupboard essentials:
200ml whole milk
1 tablespoon honey (or maple syrup
    if serving to baby under 1 year)
1 teaspoon vanilla extract

Mix the semolina with a splash of milk so that it makes a paste.

Put the rest of the milk and the orange juice in a pan and bring
to a gentle simmer.

Whisk the semolina slowly into the milk mixture and cook for 5 minutes,
whisking frequently, then remove from the heat.

Add the remaining ingredients and leave to cool.

Beat with an electric whisk until smooth.

Serve in small dishes and garnish with some orange or lemon zest.

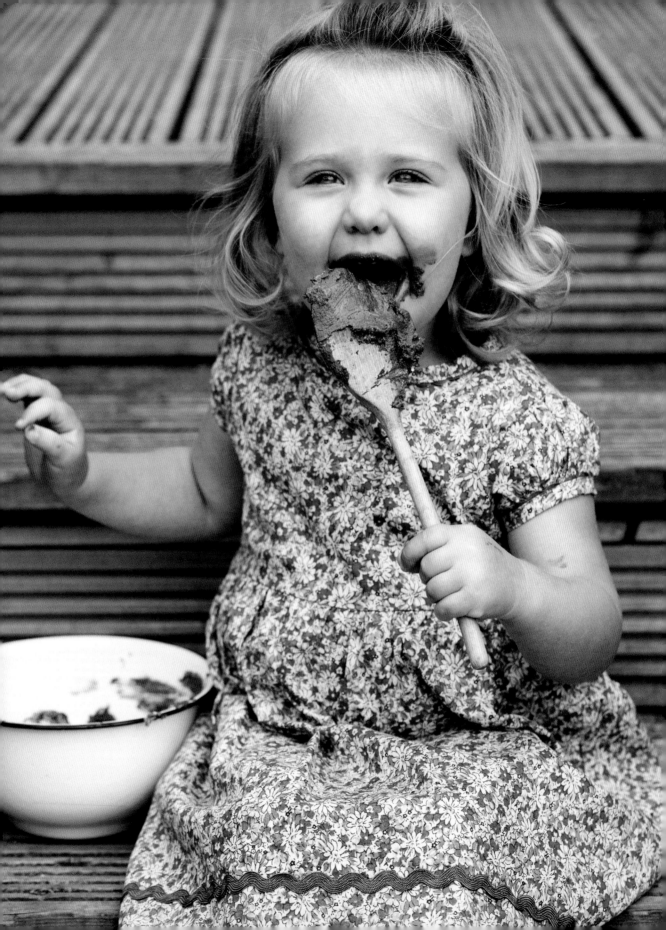

CHOCOLATE RICOTTA PUDDING

Preparation time: 5 minutes
Makes: 8 espresso-size cups

To buy:
2 x 250g tubs of ricotta
4 heaped tablespoons cocoa powder
4 tablespoons melted dark chocolate

Store-cupboard essentials:
4 tablespoons honey (or maple syrup
    if serving to baby under 1 year)
a handful of chopped pistachio nuts
    (optional)

Mix all the ingredients together in a bowl, except the pistachios, until smooth, using an electric whisk.

Divide equally between your espresso cups and serve.

Garnish with pistachio nuts, if you like.

Tips: For something a bit different, try crumbling an amaretti biscuit or digestive biscuit at the bottom of the pudding or serving with stewed fruit.

This can be refrigerated for 2-3 days. Bring to room temperature before serving.

This recipe is perhaps best kept as a treat!

BAKED ROASTED FRUIT

Preparation time: 5 minutes
Cooking time: 30 minutes
Makes: 1-2 pieces of fruit per person

To buy:
fruit of your choice

Store-cupboard essentials:
butter, melted, for drizzling
brown sugar or honey, for drizzling (avoid
   honey if serving to baby under 1 year)

Preheat the oven to 180°C/gas 4.

Cut the fruit in half and place on a baking sheet.

Scoop out any seeds or stones.

Drizzle each piece of fruit with with a little melted butter and honey
or brown sugar.

Top with your choice of sprinkles, nuts or seeds.

Bake in the oven for 30 minutes.

Finish with a dollop of cream, yoghurt or mascarpone.

Combinations:
♦ Baked apple slices with honey and cinnamon
♦ Baked peaches with mascarpone and toasted almonds
♦ Baked apricots with orange, honey and thyme
♦ Baked pears with maple syrup, raspberries and walnuts
♦ Baked plums with honey, yoghurt and coconut

Toppings
Nuts, seeds, walnuts, coconut, raspberries, mascarpone, Greek yoghurt, cinnamon, thyme, lavender.

BASIC COOKIES

Preparation time: 15 minutes
Chilling time: 30 minutes
Cooking time: 10–12 minutes
Makes: 12–16

To buy:
50g cornflour
100g icing sugar

**Variations (add one
of the following):**
♦ zest of 1 lemon or orange
♦ 40g chopped hazelnuts
♦ 2 teaspoons ground ginger

Store-cupboard essentials:
200g plain flour
180g butter, at room temperature
1 teaspoon baking powder

Preheat your oven to 180°C/gas 4.

Line a baking tray with a sheet of baking paper.

Place all the ingredients in a blender and mix
to a soft dough.

Roll into a long sausage shape and wrap in clingfilm.

Place in the fridge for a good half hour so it
becomes firm.

Slice into even discs about 1cm thick, or roll out
and cut into shapes.

Place evenly apart on a your baking tray, allowing
room for them to spread a little.

Bake for 10-12 minutes, or until golden brown.

Tips: If you can't get hold of cornflour you can use
a total of 250g plain flour.

Top the cookies with chopped nuts or dried fruit
of your choice before baking.

SWEET POTATO COOKIES

Preparation time: 15 minutes
Cooking time: 10–12 minutes
Makes: 10–12

To buy:

1 medium sweet potato, roasted
100g ground almonds
100g unsweetened desiccated coconut
1 tablespoon coconut oil, melted
a handful of chocolate chips

Store-cupboard essentials:

½ teaspoon bicarbonate of soda
1 tablespoon ground cinnamon
½ teaspoon sea salt
2 tablespoons honey (or maple syrup
   if serving to baby under 1 year)
2 teaspoons vanilla extract
1 egg
a handful of chopped nuts of your choice

Preheat the oven to 180°C/gas 4.

Blitz the cooked sweet potato to a purée using a stick blender or pot attachment.

Combine the dry ingredients in a small bowl – ground almonds, coconut, bicarbonate of soda, cinnamon and salt (if making for toddlers and adults only).

Mix the sweet potato, coconut oil, honey, vanilla extract and egg together.

Fold the dry ingredients into the wet ingredients and stir in the chopped nuts and choc chips. If the mixture seems dry, add another egg yolk.

Scoop balls of the mixture on to a lined baking tray and flatten to form round cookies – they will not spread on their own.

Bake for 10–12 minutes and leave to cool on the tray.

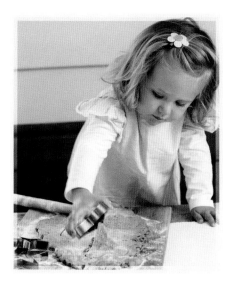

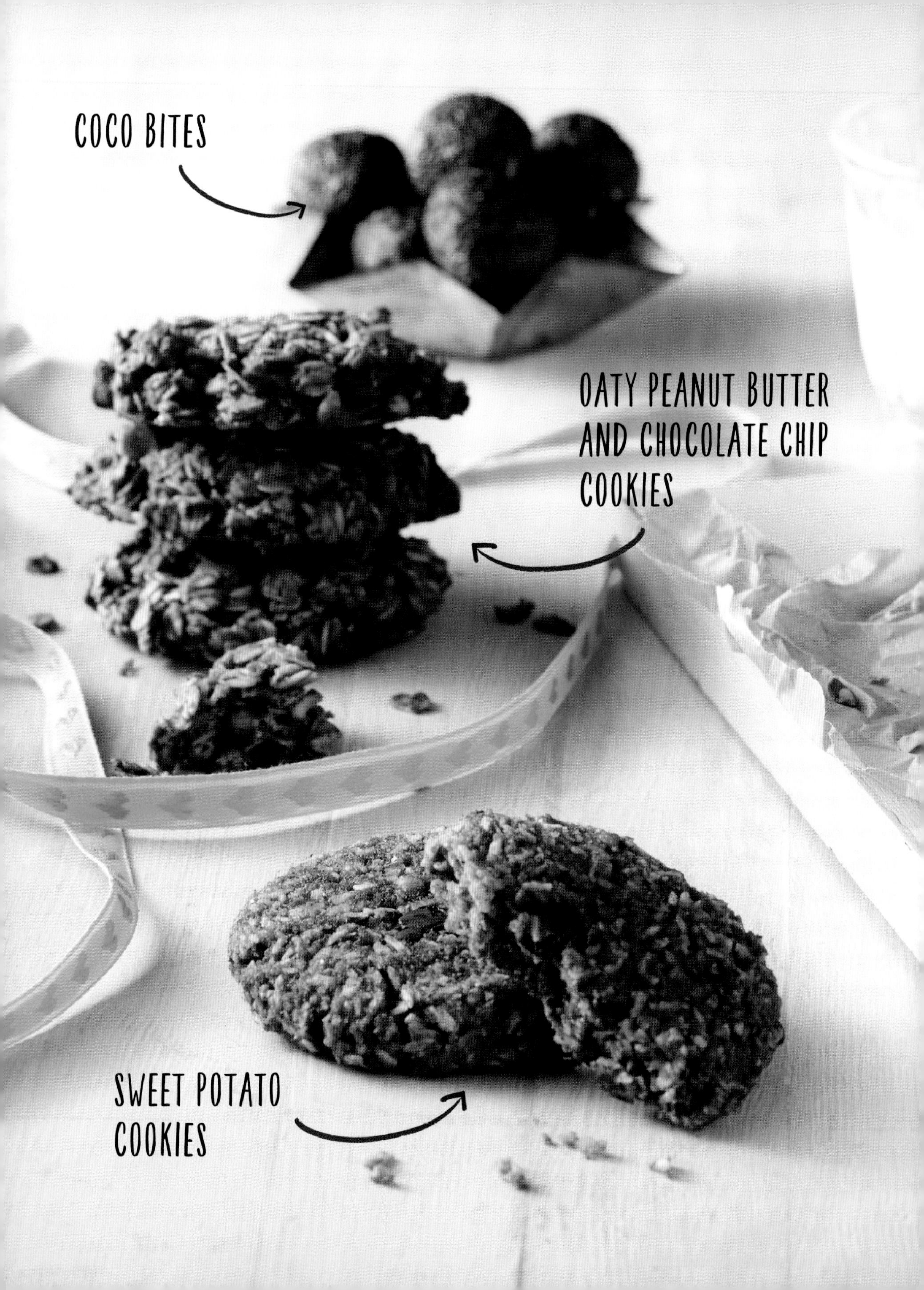

COCO BITES

OATY PEANUT BUTTER
AND CHOCOLATE CHIP
COOKIES

SWEET POTATO
COOKIES

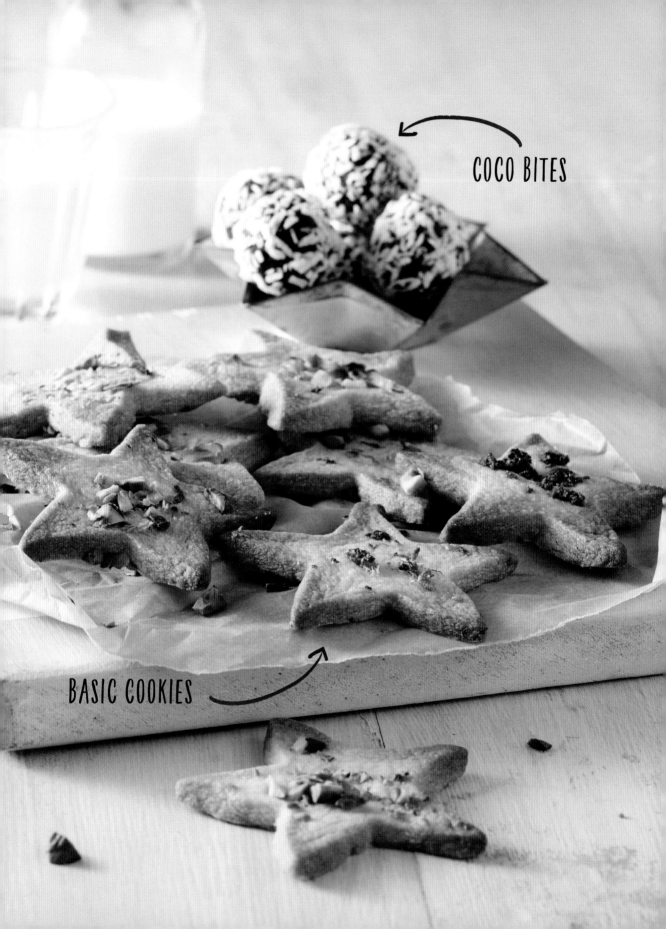

COCO BITES

BASIC COOKIES

OATY PEANUT BUTTER AND CHOCOLATE CHIP COOKIES

Preparation time: 5 minutes
Cooking time: 10–12 minutes
Makes: 8–10

To buy:
1 tablespoon crunchy peanut butter
a handful of dark chocolate chips

Store-cupboard essentials:
150g oats
80g honey (or maple syrup if serving
   to baby under 1 year)
25g butter, melted
1 egg
½ teaspoon bicarbonate of soda
½ teaspoon vanilla extract

Preheat the oven to 180°C/gas 4.

Mix all the ingredients together and leave for 5-10 minutes for the oats to absorb the egg mixture.

Dollop a tablespoon of the mixture at a time on to a baking tray lined with parchment paper. Leave space between each cookie.

Bake for 10-12 minutes, until golden brown. It is important to be patient and let the cookies cool before eating, as they are soft and will fall apart if eaten too soon.

Tip: You can substitute any nuts or dried fruits for the choc chips and peanut butter.

COCO BITES

Preparation time: 10 minutes
Chilling time: 15 minutes
Freezing time: 20 minutes
Makes: approx. 14

To buy:

1 ripe banana

6 tablespoons cocoa powder

2 handfuls of unsweetened dessicated
   coconut, plus extra for rolling

2 tablespoons coconut oil, melted

Store-cupboard essentials:

2 tablespoons pure maple syrup
   (or other liquid sweetener)

½ teaspoon vanilla extract

½ teaspoon ground cinnamon

Mash the banana well and place in a large mixing bowl.

Mix all the remaining ingredients together until well combined.

Chill in the fridge for 15 minutes for the mixture to firm up.

Line a baking sheet with parchment paper or a non-stick mat.

Roll the mixture into walnut-size balls and place on the tray. Roll half in the dessicated coconut and leave half plain.

Freeze for approximately 20 minutes, or until the balls are firm.

Store in the freezer until ready to enjoy. They will soften at room temperature – take them out about 10–15 minutes before you need them.

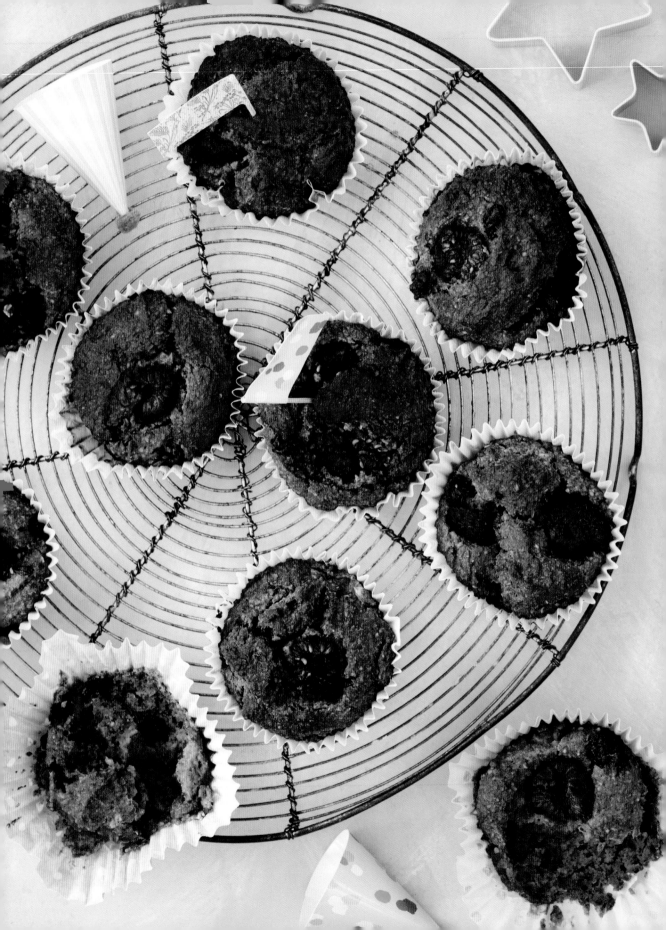

GRAB-AND-GO OAT MUFFINS

Preparation time: 10 minutes
Cooking time: 30–40 minutes
Makes: 24 mini or 12 big muffins

To buy:
80g ground almonds
80g super seeds (sunflower,
 pumpkin, flax, chia or hemp)
1 x small tub of yoghurt (100g)
 (we used Greek, but any full-fat
 yoghurt will do)
2 ripe bananas, peeled
a handful of frozen or fresh
 raspberries
a handful of raisins

Store-cupboard essentials:
80g oats
1½ teaspoons baking powder
1 teaspoon ground cinnamon
4 tablespoons maple syrup or
 honey (avoid honey if serving
 to baby under 1 year)
olive oil

Preheat your oven to 180°C/gas 4.

Blend the oats, ground almonds and seeds in a stick blender pot attachment.

Add the other ingredients, apart from the raspberries and raisins, and blitz until smooth.

Transfer to a mixing bowl and gently stir in the raspberries and raisins.

Grease a muffin tin with a little oil and fill each cup with the mixture to just about the top.

Bake in the middle of the oven for 30–40 minutes, until a skewer inserted into the centre of a muffin comes out clean.

Cool before enjoying.

Tip: Try using a handful of blueberries or apricots, or a grated apple, carrot or courgette instead of the raspberries and raisins.

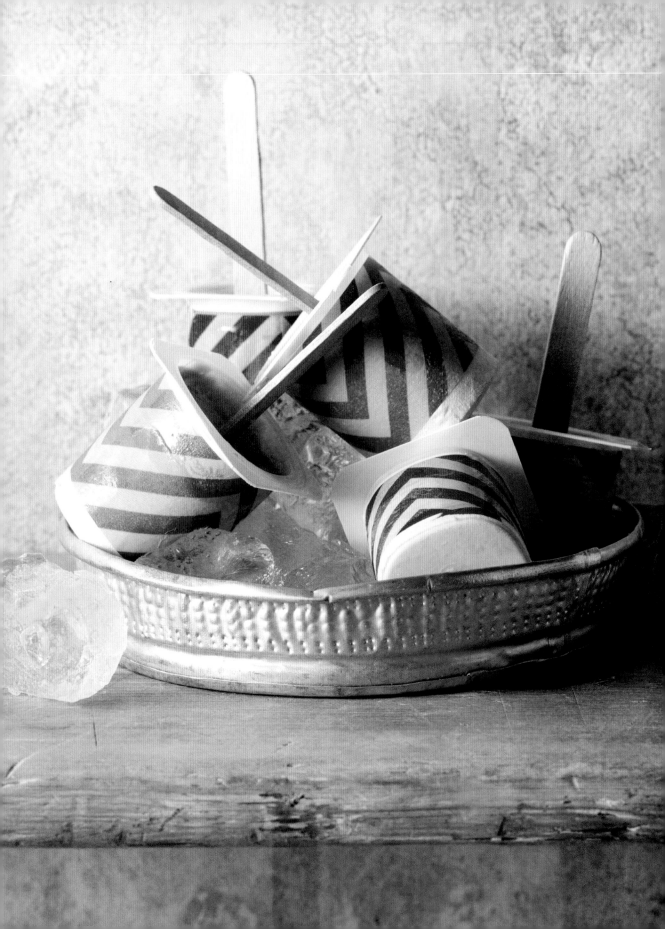

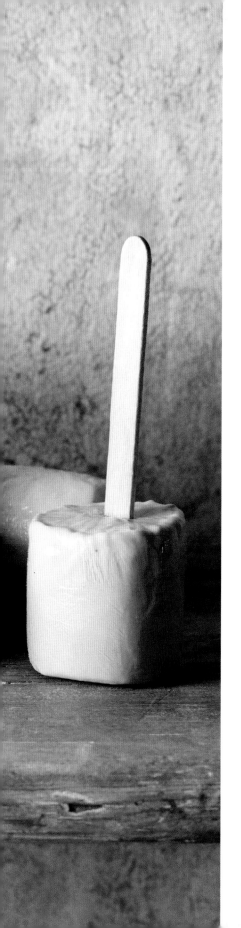

MINI FROZEN YOGHURT POTS

Preparation time: 2 minutes
Freezing time: 3–4 hours
Serves: 4

To buy:
4 mini yoghurts, such as Petits Filous
wooden lolly sticks

Pierce the lid of the yoghurt pot with the wooden stick, making sure it stands up straight.

Freeze for 3-4 hours, or until frozen.

Peel off the lid of the yoghurt pot, then pop the frozen yoghurt lolly out of its container and enjoy.

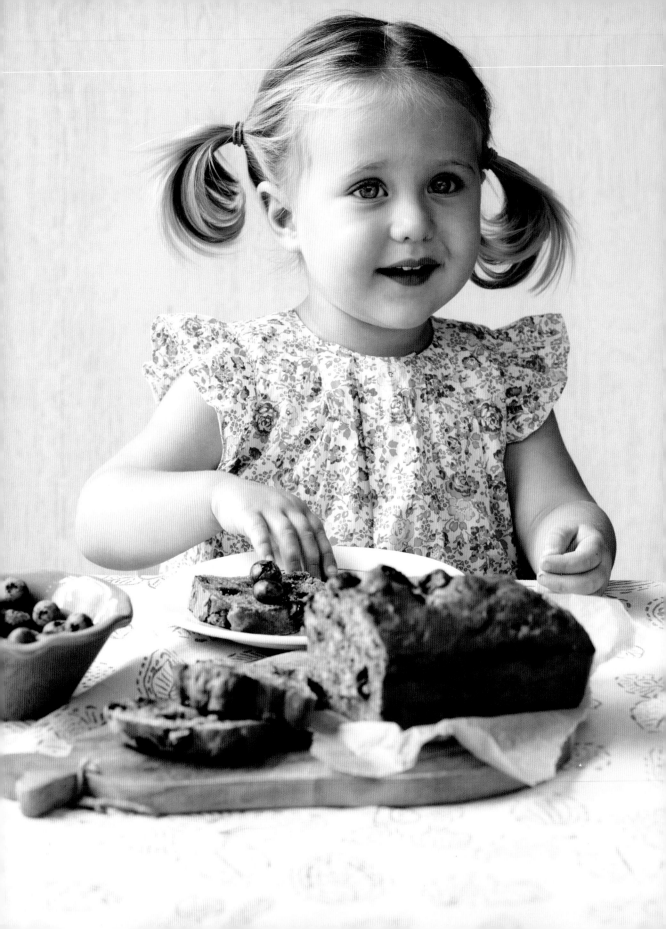

BLUEBERRY BANANA BREAD

Preparation time: 10 minutes
Cooking time: 50–60 minutes
Serves: 6

To buy:
3 bananas, mashed
120g wholewheat flour
2 handfuls of fresh
   blueberries

Store-cupboard essentials:
2 eggs
2 tablespoons olive oil
2 tablespoons honey (avoid serving
   to baby under 1 year)
1 teaspoon vanilla extract
50g plain flour
1½ teaspoons baking powder
¼ teaspoon bicarbonate of soda
½ teaspoon ground cinnamon

Preheat your oven to 180°C/gas 4.

Grease and line a loaf tin and set aside.

Mix in the bananas, eggs, oil, honey and vanilla extract.

Add your dry ingredients – both flours, baking powder, bicarbonate of soda and cinnamon – and mix until well combined.

Stir in the blueberries.

Pour into your loaf tin and bake for 50–60 minutes.

Check if the bread is cooked – it's ready when a skewer inserted into the centre comes out clean.

Leave to cool completely before tucking in.

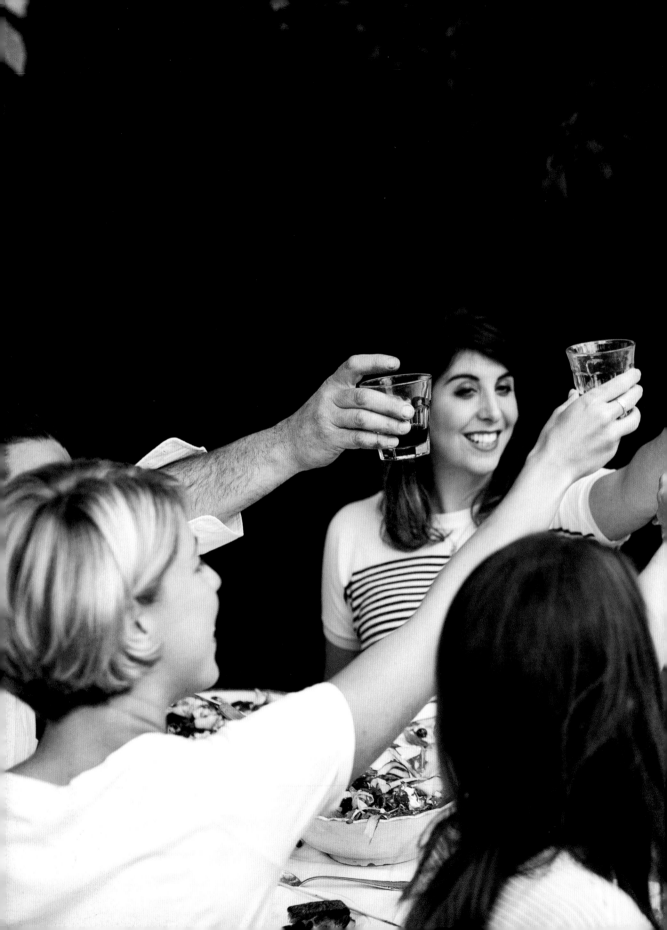

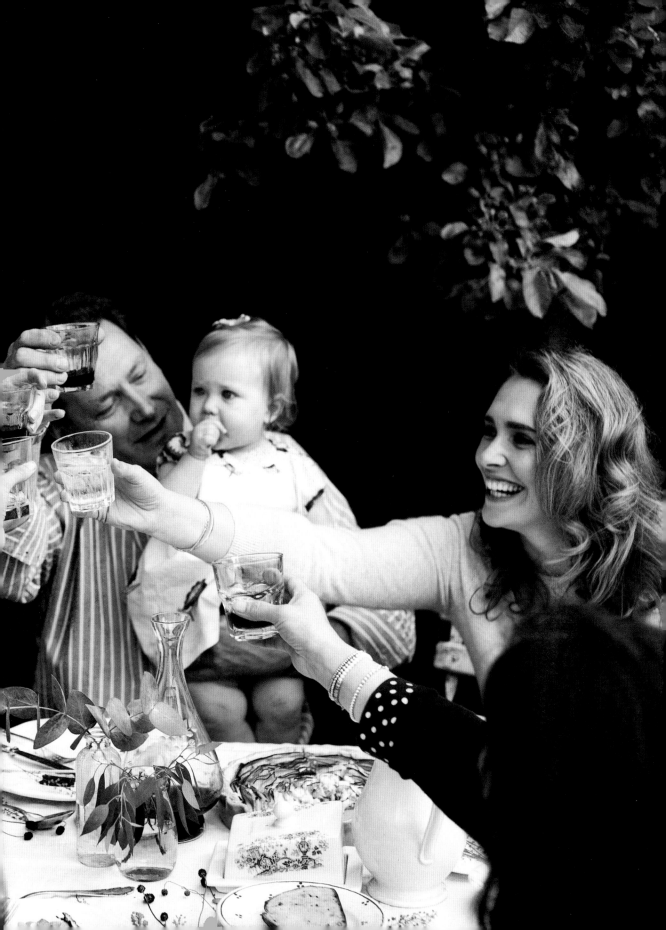

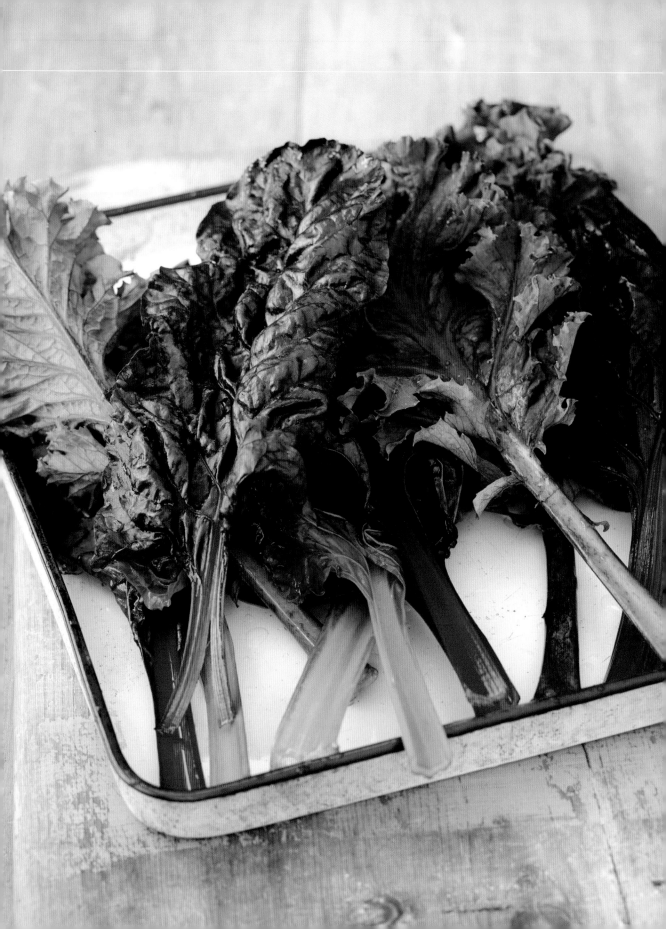

NUTRIENTS EVERY CHILD NEEDS AND WHY

Here is a list of key nutrients that every child should have, with the reasons why. Breast-fed or formula-fed babies will receive these nutrients from their milk until 6 months, and then gradually, as weaning starts to substitute milk from 6–12 months, food will become the main source of these nutrients.

Protein

- For growth.
- Helps repair all body tissues.
- Helps produce enzymes that control many body functions, e.g. nervous-system function.

....

Good sources of protein:
- Meat
- Fish
- Eggs
- Dairy products
- Beans and pulses
- Tofu
- Nuts and seeds

Zinc

- Our bodies require zinc for many different things, one of its main roles being in the metabolism of several nutrients in the body.
- Aids immune-system function, cell protection and bone health. Given its variety of uses in the body, zinc deficiency can have several adverse effects on a baby's growth and general health.

....

Good sources of zinc:
- Meat (beef, pork)
- Wholegrains (wholemeal wheat flour)
- Dairy products (cheese)
- Beans and pulses (red kidney beans)
- Nuts and seeds (almonds, peanuts, sunflower seeds)

....

Disclaimer: Ingredient information taken from McCance and Widdowson's 2015 ingredient database, and all health claims for referenced nutrients are approved on the EU register of nutrition and health claims.

Vitamin D

- Helps the absorption of calcium, one of the minerals that make up our bones and teeth.
- Important for immune system function and muscle function.

Useful information: We should be getting most of our vitamin D from sunlight exposure; however, babies and children are spending less time outdoors, and at certain times of the year, when our skin isn't able to make vitamin D from sunlight, it is important to understand the food sources of vitamin D and to make sure these foods are included in the diet.

Vitamin D deficiency is also common in pregnant and breastfeeding women, so including lots of food sources of vitamin D into the diet of these groups is equally important and can impact your baby.

Vitamin D deficiency can result in the development of rickets in children, which is the softening of bone, resulting in a bow-legged appearance.

Good sources of vitamin D:
- Found almost exclusively in fish (e.g. salmon)
- Eggs (the yolks)
- Also fortified in breakfast cereals and some fortified spreads – make sure you are avoiding any breakfast cereals with added sugar, salt or flavourings

Iron

- Important for cognitive, metabolic and immune function.
- Aids red blood cell and haemoglobin production. Haemoglobin carries oxygen around the body, which in turns helps to prevent us feeling tired.

Useful information: Iron deficiency anaemia can occur in babies and children who do not get enough iron; they will appear pale and tired and some appetite may be lost. The long-term effects of iron deficiency impact on cognitive function and behaviour. Too much iron, however, could also be harmful, which is why it is better to get iron from food sources rather than supplements, unless iron deficiency has been diagnosed and supplements are used as a treatment.

Good sources of iron:
- Certain meats and fish (beef, pork, anchovies). Iron from animal sources is more easily absorbed than iron from plant sources, so try to mix it up and get both in
- Eggs
- Fortified breakfast cereals – again, try to avoid any with added sugar, salt or flavourings
- Certain beans (kidney beans, black-eyed beans, red lentils)
- Dark green leafy vegetables (spinach).
- Nuts (cashews)
- Dried apricots
- Wheat flour – wheat flour in the UK has to be fortified with iron by law

Calcium

- An important mineral that makes up our bones and teeth.
- Helps our nervous system function.
- Helps with blood clotting and muscle function.
- Important for metabolic function (the process by which our bodies extract energy and nutrients from foods).

Useful information: Having enough calcium is particularly important in babies and young children, as bone growth is happening at such a fast rate. Insufficient calcium can, like vitamin D deficiency, also lead to the development of rickets.

Good sources of calcium:
- Milk
- Other dairy products such as yoghurt
- Fortified soya, nut and oat milks
- Some pulses, such as chickpeas
- Some nuts and seeds (almonds, Brazil nuts, sesame seeds)
- Dark green leafy vegetables (spinach and kale)
- Wheat flour and products made with wheat flour – wheat flour in the UK has to be fortified with calcium by law

PRODUCTS WE LOVE...

Baby bag

As mums we spent AGES looking for the best nappy/baby bag. It HAD to be practical (i.e. it needed to fit a lot in, with compartments and practical spaces), but we really wanted it to look nice too. We decided that a backpack is the ideal solution for keeping your hands free (especially with more than one baby!). We absolutely love Tiba + Marl (www.tibaandmarl.com), who do a huge range of glam mummy bags at affordable prices.

Béaba and Oxo

Brilliant travel containers for taking your Pick 'n' Mix Cubes with you when you're on the go. (www.beaba.com and www.oxouk.com)

Books

We are bringing our kids up to be bilingual, so we love any books with script in both languages. Any exposure to another language is brilliant for kids, so check out www.little-linguist.co.uk.

Also, these books are a fab invention – as their name suggests, indestructibles (www.indestructiblesinc.com) can be thrown in water, chewed or stretched and they will still remain in one piece!

Italian delis

Our fave is the online store (www.nifeislife.com), for brilliant fresh produce delivered to your door.

Merino wool sleep sacks

Yes, expensive, but worth every penny (and if you manage to score one in the sale . . . bingo! This is the only sleep sack I used/you need. It lasted from birth until my little one went into a big bed with proper PJs, and is all you need in summer and winter. Worth every penny! (www.bambinomerino.com)

Mini Boden

We love so much of Mini Boden's collections (www.boden.co.uk) . . . always a struggle to choose, as there's so much we want!

Mini First Aid

A nationwide course for parents or guardians that we would thoroughly recommend. It's only a 2-hour course and one that we think every parent should do. It teaches you basic knowledge of how to deal with choking and other common worries such as burns, cuts and illness. Visit www.minifirstaid.co.uk to find a course near you.

Moulin Roty

So, so, so much we want, from the softest teddies to gorgeous school satchels (www. moulinroty.com).

No-mess paints

We love doing creative sessions with our girls, but paints can be a real faff, especially if the kids don't have a long attention span. Maped Color'Peps Smoothy Gel Crayons and PlayColour Solid Paint Sticks are brilliant, as they look like paints, beautifully vibrant and thick, but they write like crayons, avoiding a scary mess!

RICE kids' crockery

Gorgeous designs, hardwearing, and the best way to glam up your kids' meals (www. ricebyrice.com).

Teething beads

We love Coo CaChoo, an independent supplier of teething beads. Made to order and in your preferred colours, their creations are beads for mum and baby. Such cute designs (www.facebook.com/CooCaChooCreations).

The Wee Department Store

The ultimate online store for kids' clothes. When getting to the shops is a challenge, it's the best retail therapy right from your sofa. We love clothes with cute details for kiddies, and there is always something unique. (www. theweedepartmentstore.co.uk)

Toys and games

We love Hape and Djeco toys and games – such innovative ideas, and Djeco does loads of fabulous creative ideas for toddlers and older kids too. (www.hapetoys.com and www. djeco.com)

Your equipment essentials

We love our 30cm oval almond Le Creuset cast iron pan as our . . . 4 in 1 delight (www.lecreuset. co.uk). As for our stick blender . . . we have a good ol' Kenwood Tri Blade hand blender with pot attachment (www.kenwoodworld.com).

GRAZIE MILLE...

The biggest thanks to our mum, for all her help and inspiration with this book – you are like another sister to us and you can never know how much we value you and how much you inspire us all. Always at our side at a drop of a hat, you are the best! Also thanks to our dad, who is getting more used to our crazy schedules!

To our sister Romina, thanks for all your help with the book and for being the best team leader to all your nieces. Always willing to roll up your sleeves and get stuck into baby madness – we love you so much.

To our husbands Dan and O. E., we know you think we are crazy with everything we do while trying to raise our kids, Fiamma, Serafina and Fiorenza, but your love, support and encouragement mean everything to us.

A massive thank you to our wonderful editor Lindsey Evans, who once again believed in our vision for this book and made it happen, always with a smile on her face while dealing with a whole Italian family's conflicting opinions. And to our agent, Jess Stone, for believing in us and encouraging us to stay true to ourselves. You are a constant support and someone we can always trust to give the best advice.

Jenni, what can we say; you've understood us sisters and our brand from the moment you started working with us. Your design ideas are always spot on and gorgeous and you have helped shape this book into what it has become . . . thanks for listening to us and nailing it every single time. As always it has been amazing to work with you and we hope to do so many more times . . . if you can still put up with us!

A big shout-out to our photoshoot group: Frankie, Danielle and Ted – whose patience and amazing vision during our crazy shoot days were out of this world. Thanks for helping to make the book look so wonderful.

A million thank-yous to all the mums who have supported the book, giving us feedback and honest opinions: Becca, Claire, Jules, Kate, Katherine, Lisa, Lizzie, Lucy, Mel, Sue and NCT mums. You were the best guinea pigs, and your comments and critiques were so appreciated – we could not have done it without you. Also thanks for letting us snap some pics of your gorgeous children to include in the book. Special thanks go to our good friends Claudine, who has helped give us so much wonderful recipe inspiration over the years, and Jules, who has been an amazing support on so many levels - as a mum, babysitter and undercover editor!

And finally to the Sherborne businesses who helped support our shoot. Biggest thanks to the amazing Mike at Castle Garden Centre, who provided such a wonderful location, never questioning our random requests for props and equipment! Thanks also to all the shops that supported the shoot – Ginger & Pickles, Ally at Butterfly Bright, The Circus, and Adrian and family at Market Town Garden (the lovely fruit and veg shop on Cheap Street).

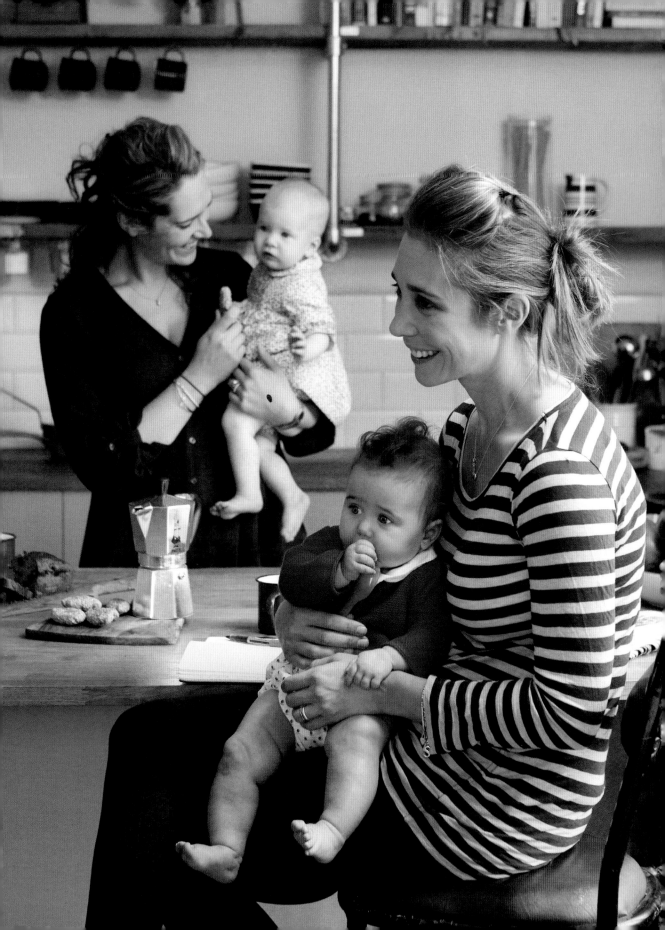

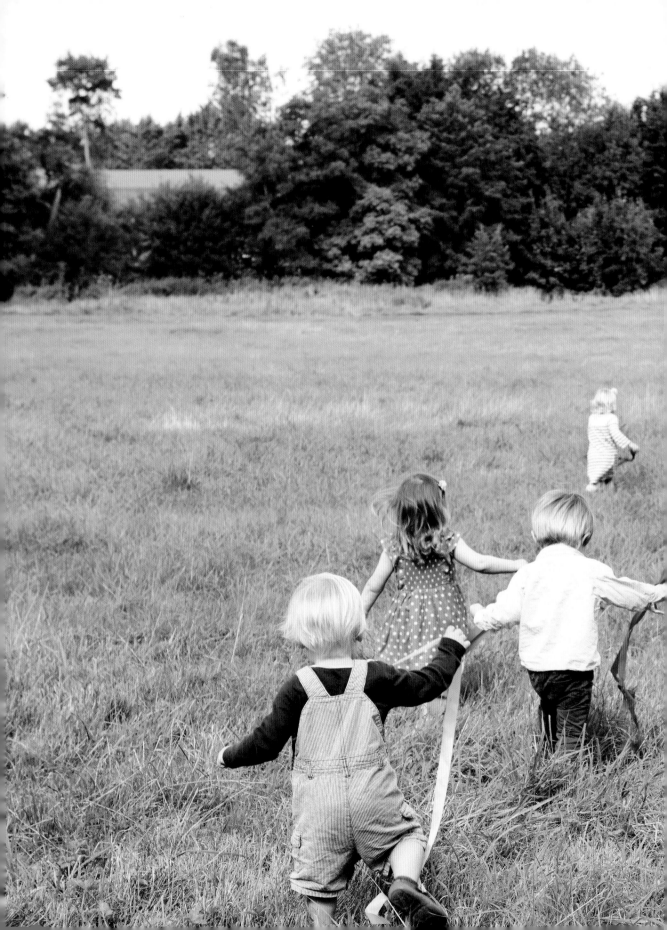

We would love to hear from you – do send us pictures of your recipe creations, your baby weaning stories or tales of stubborn toddlers and tag us!

🌐   www.thechiappas.com

▶️ **You Tube**   www.youtube.com/TheChiappaSisters

🐦   @theChiappas

f   TheChiappas

📷   @theChiappas

INDEX